I0758837

Vagus Nerve

Self-healing Techniques for Stress, Anxiety, Depression, Panic Attacks. ADHD, Chronic Illness and Inflammation. Relax Your Nervous System and Heal Your Body Through Mind-Gut Connection

By Albert Dales

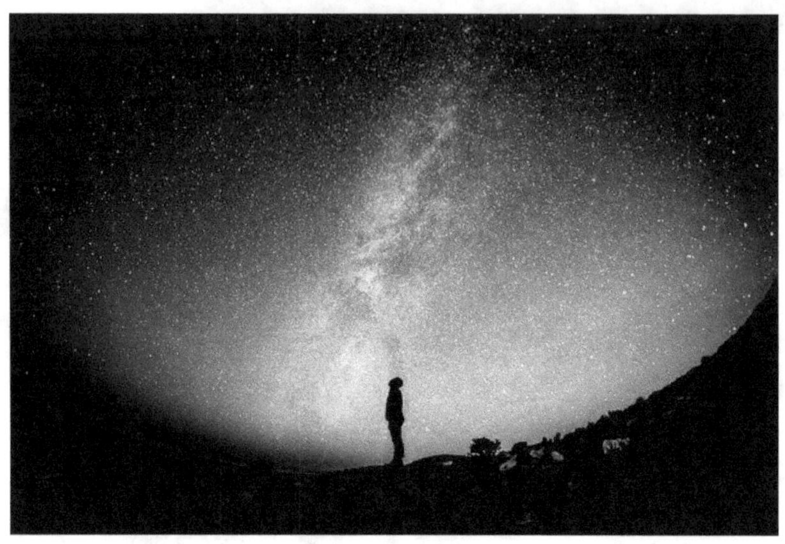

© **Copyright 2019 by Albert Dales - All rights reserved.**

The content contained within this book may not be reproduced, duplicated or transmitted without direct written permission from the author or the publisher.

Under no circumstances will any blame or legal responsibility be held against the publisher, or author, for any damages, reparation, or monetary loss due to the information contained within this book. Either directly or indirectly.

Legal Notice:

This book is copyright protected. This book is only for personal use. You cannot amend, distribute, sell, use, quote or paraphrase any part, or the content within this book, without the consent of the author or publisher.

Disclaimer Notice:

Please note the information contained within this document is for educational and entertainment purposes only. All effort has been executed to present accurate, up to date, and reliable, complete information. No warranties of any kind are declared or implied. Readers acknowledge that the author is not engaging in the rendering of legal, financial, medical or professional advice. The content within this book has been derived from various sources. Please consult a licensed professional before attempting any techniques outlined in this book.

By reading this document, the reader agrees that under no circumstances is the author responsible for any losses, direct or indirect, which are incurred as a result of the use of the information contained within this document, including, but not limited to, — errors, omissions, or inaccuracies.

Table of Contents

Introduction

Congratulations on purchasing Vagus Nerve: Self-healing Techniques for Stress, Anxiety, Depression, Panic Attacks. ADHD, Chronic Illness and Inflammation. Relax Your Nervous System and Heal Your Body Through Mind-Gut Connection and thank you for doing so.

If you are reading this book it is because you are keen on learning more about how you can improve your overall health and wellbeing by improving your understanding of how the body works. In particular, your understanding of the nervous system will enable you to gain a deeper insight into the way your body is able to process many of the situations that it encounters on a daily basis.

The vagus nerve is one, if not, the most important neural network in the human body. It controls a number of systems which are vital to the overall functioning of the body's essential biological functions. That means that if the vagus nerve does not perform up to its optimal capabilities, the effects on the overall functioning of the body can be significant. Hence, there is a great need for everyone to understand how it works, what it does and what can be done to ensure that it functions up to its full potential.

Moreover, the vagus nerve is not fully understood. Its incredible power hasn't been fully understood until recently. Modern research has revealed the importance of this nerve and the need for its care. This has given way to a score of approaches with the aim to keep the vagus nerve in peak performance. In this book, we will discuss these approaches as a means of ensuring that we are able to maintain optimal health and wellbeing, both of the vagus nerve itself, and by extension, the body systems that it controls.

This book has been written with the intent to inform the general public on this topic. So, even a novice in the topic of the nervous system will be able to make the most of this important issue. After all, we are not here to provide complex information; rather, our intent is to provide you with information you won't easily find anywhere else.

As such, this book has been written with the aim of allowing anyone who is interested in learning about the topic the opportunity to do so in plain language. This book isn't an attempt at trying to sound smart; it is an exercise in helping the average individual learn as much as they can in a clear and concise manner. That means that we are going to be getting down to the meat and potatoes of this topic straight from the get-go.

This is an important consideration especially since the vagus nerve is indeed the body's main control module. Also, given the fact that we tend to know very little about it, we end up ignoring its relevance in our overall health and wellbeing. When we understand what this nerve does in our body, we are able to make a conscious choice to ensure its health. In doing so, we can keep a good level of physical wellbeing.

It should also be noted that our emotions also play a key role in maintaining the health of the vagus nerve. So, we need to be keen on understanding how we can address our emotional life in benefit of our overall body's performance. With this book, you will be able to get a working knowledge of how this can be achieved. It really is possible however unlikely it may seem.

Best of all, the information provided herein is intended to help you get off the ground and into a great physical condition. So, let's jump right on in and discuss how you can use the information we will discuss throughout to improve your overall quality of life. You will surely find that improving your physical health and emotional wellbeing isn't nearly as complicated as you might have thought. Indeed, you will have the power and the knowledge you need to improve your quality of life by the end of this book.

So, thank you once again for taking the time to read this book. We are certain that you will find the information contained herein to be both useful and informative. And don't worry if you haven't heard much about the topic. The fact is that the research discussed throughout this book is quite new. Thus, it hasn't quite made its way into the mainstream media. Over the next few years, you can expect more and more information to trickle its way into the mainstream. In the meantime, you have a primer at hand. In a manner of speaking, you are getting a look at the full movie well before it premieres at the cinema. So, sit back and enjoy the topic at hand. We do hope it will help you achieve a healthier version of yourself and your loved ones.

Let's get started!

PART I: THE NERVOUS SYSTEM

Chapter 1: The Central Nervous System

The starting point in this book is a discussion on the Central Nervous System (CNS). The CNS is perhaps the single most important component of the entire human body. It is the control center of the entire body's functioning. It essentially controls everything that happens throughout the body. As such, there is no function that is not controlled, one way or another, by the nervous system.

Generally speaking, the CNS is comprised of the brain and the main control unit and the spinal cord. The spinal cord then branches out into the millions of individual nerves that control the information sent from the brain and into each body component.

It is safe to say that without the CNS and its neural network, none of what we do would be possible. Think about a person who has been in an accident. If the suffer significant trauma to the brain, or perhaps the spinal cord, they may lose control over certain body parts. For instance, a severed spinal cord at the base of the neck will essentially mean that a person can be completely paralyzed from the neck down.

However, despite the loss of body movement, it is still possible for the Autonomic Nervous System (ANS) to function thereby maintaining essential body functions such as breathing, digestion, and blood flow. While we will discuss the ANS later on, it is worth mentioning that significant trauma to the brain and spinal cord does not necessarily mean a death sentence for the sufferer. In fact, modern science has made great advancements in the regeneration of the nervous system to the point where once paralyzed individuals are now able to regain much of their body's original functions.

Parts of the CNS

The CNS mainly consists of two parts, the brain, and the spinal cord. So, let's take a look at what each one of these parts does and how they are comprised.

The brain

The main processing unit of the entire CNS is the brain. The brain houses cells called neurons. Neurons are the cells which are responsible for relaying information back and forth. As such, the brain serves as one immense messaging center. Millions of messages are relayed at any given moment. These messages control everything from voluntary movements, such as reaching out for a cup of coffee, to all of the involuntary movements such as breathing. These involuntary functions are vital. After all, if you stop breathing, you would die.

The brain is also believed to control thoughts and emotions. While mythological and cultural beliefs contend that emotions are housed in specific organs (for example love is believed to reside in the heart) the fact of the matter is that emotions are a psychological response to the stimuli around us.

The brain mainly consists of four parts:

- The frontal lobe
- The temporal lobe
- The parietal lobe
- The occipital lobe

The sum of these four lobes is known as the cerebrum. In addition, the brain is divided into two hemispheres.

While there is much research still ongoing, much of the brain's overall functioning remains a mystery. Of course, science has decoded the brain's main workings, but it is the finer points of the brain which we still struggle to comprehend. For instance, the nature of thought, which is believed to be housed in the brain, largely remains unclear.

That being said, the various parts of the brain are in charge of various functions. So, it is certainly worth digging deeper into them.

The frontal lobe is responsible for the majority of human cognitive skills such as emotional expression, memory, linguistic skills, problem-solving abilities, and even sexual behavior. It is indeed one of the most important parts of the brain for modern homo sapiens.

The temporal lobe is in charge of managing key features such as language, speech and comprehension skills. A significant lesion to the temporal lobe may leave the sufferer unable to communicate appropriately. As such, blows to the head may result in impaired cognitive abilities.

The parietal lobe can be found behind the frontal lobe. Its main function is the processing of sensory input, that is, information that enters from the five senses. This information is decoded by the parietal lobe and transformed into usable knowledge that the individual can then use as a part of daily life.

The occipital lobe is found at the back of the head. Its main purpose is to process visual information. As such, this information is taken from visual input (the eyes) and then transformed into working data which is perceived by the mind as a visual representation of stimuli. A good example of this is how light is decoded by the brain to reveal the color.

The spinal cord

The spine is one of the distinguishing characteristics of homo sapiens. Firstly, humans are able to walk upright. While this trait is not exclusive to humans, it is very uncommon in nature. Only a handful of mammals are capable of walking upright. As a result, the spine enables the human body to maintain its upright structure.

Furthermore, the spine is also the hub for the entire neural network that runs throughout the body. This is why lesions to the spine may lead to severe disruption of bodily functions. In addition, the spine is also divided into parts that govern the functioning and movement of the body.

The bones which make up the spine are called vertebrae. Each vertebra has a form of a disc. Each disc is insulated with a gelatin-like substance. This substance can wear down over time. When this happens, individual nerves may get caught in between two vertebrae. This may cause excruciating pain, issues with mobility or even paralysis. In general, such situations may be remedied by surgery though the outcome isn't always assured.

The junction at which the brain is joined to the spinal cord is known as the brain stem. This is the most sensitive part of the CNS as the entire neural network passes through this section. As such, a serious injury to the neck could prove catastrophic to an individual.

The layers which cover the brain and the spinal cord are known as meninges. These layers serve as insulation so that the brain and spinal cord are isolated from bacteria and infection. Also, deep inside the spine is the spinal fluid. This fluid is responsible for nourishing the spine and the brain.

Lastly, it should be mentioned that proper blood flow throughout the CNS is vital in order to ensure proper functioning. If insufficient amounts of oxygen circulate in the blood, potential damage can be sustained. If the supply of oxygen is cut off completely, irreversible damage may be caused to the CNS leading the sufferer to experience anything from cognitive dysfunction to physical limitations.

Chapter 2: The role of nerves in the CNS

The CNS communicates with the entire body through an intricate network of nerves. As such, nerves as thread-like membranes that run through every part of the body. This is the means of communication that the body maintains with individual body parts.

Here is a good example of how this communication takes place.

One of the most important responses that the CNS produces is pain. Pain is the body's natural way of signaling that there is a potentially destructive situation underway. For instance, a person has stubbed their toe on their coffee table. The blow is recorded by the nerve receptors in the toe. The sensation is relayed through the nerves and up to the brain. The brain then decodes the information and sends back a signal indicating that this is pain. The toe then receives the information and decides that this is not good. As a result, the individual feels tremendous pain which is meant to be taken as a signal of damage to that part of the body.

A further nervous response could be swelling in the toe. This inflammation is the body's natural way of isolating an injured body part. In a way, it is like sending the police to close off the area and ensure that help gets to where it needs to.

This entire process seems like a long one; and in reality, it is. However, it takes place in a matter of nanoseconds. The body's processing capabilities far exceed any capability that computers are currently able to display.

That being said, the CNS is made up of four main types of nerves. This is important to note as nerves are a one-size-fits-all proposition. Nerves are highly specialized so that they are able to relay the right messages as accurately as possible.

The reason for dedicated neural networks can be attributed to evolution. The evolution of the human brain required the development of specialized types of nerves, cells, and receptors. Give the fact that humans are highly complex machines, certainly much more complex when compared to other mammals, the need for specialized and dedicated neural networks becomes evident.

Cranial nerves
Cranial nerves are located within the cranium, that is, the head. These nerves are essentially dedicated to the processes

that occur within the head and are associated to the eyes, mouth, ears, nose and any other process that occurs directly within the cranium. They are highly important as they control four of the five senses. In addition, the facial muscles are the most complex muscle system in the body. Facial muscles are comprised of minuscule groups that enable humans to use their faces to express feelings and communicate non-verbally.

Furthermore, the cranial nerves process sight, sound, taste, and smell. Indeed, they are constantly working in overdrive thereby enabling a person to perceive the environment around them in the most efficient manner possible.

Central nerves

The central nerves run from the brain and down the spine. In a manner of speaking, they are the main highway from which individual side roads branch off to specific destinations. This implies that central nerves need to be the most robust nerves in the body as they must tend to thousand and thousands of messages per second. Their capability enables the body to make any number of movements simultaneously. If central nerves happen to become damaged, for example as a result of infection, then a person's motor development may become impaired.

Peripheral nerves

The periphery of the CNS is associated to the nerves which control messaging in the limbs. This is what enables, arms, legs, feet, toes, hands, and fingers to move with ease. It should be said that this neural network develops as we progress from childhood to maturity. Therefore, it is of the utmost importance for children to engage is as much physical activity as possible. A lack of physical activity during childhood may lead to decreased motor skill development.

Autonomic nerves

This neural network is the unsung hero of the human body. These nerves control the involuntary movements that keep the body alive. These nerves ensure the functioning of the heart, lungs, brain, digestive system, among other essential biological functions. Moreover, these nerves are so specialized, that they cannot be easily repaired by the body. That is why any neural damage to this particular network, such as the result of an illness like diabetes, may lead to irreversible consequences. That is why renal failure is common among diabetics much the same way that prolonged hypertension damages blood vessels, the heart muscle, and autonomic nerves.

Neurons

The last component of the CNS is known are the neuron. Neurons are cells that resemble worker bees; they do the yeoman's work of the entire nervous system in such a way that they enable to transmission of information from one part of the body to another. It is safe to say that if neurons should fail for whatever reason, the body may encounter grave complications.

In essence, neurons work on electrochemical impulses that transmit information by means of relays. So, while the nerves themselves act as a highway, the neurons in the brain work on a relay system. What this enables the brain to do is process a multitude of operations in a matter of nanoseconds. Each neuron is composed of the cell body, dendrites, and axon. The dendrites are tiny branches that receive sensory information. Then, the axon takes that sensory information and passes it on to another cell. This is a thread-like branch that enables communication among cells.

There are three main types of neurons.

- Multipolar neurons contain one axon and a number of dendrites. They are commonly found in the spinal cord and the brain. They serve to relay all sorts of information to the nerves where they need to go.
- Bipolar neurons contain a single axon and a single dendrite. These can be seen in the retina of the eye, in

the nose (olfactory cells) and in the inner ear. These are highly specialized neurons.

- Unipolar neurons focus on one type of process throughout the body. This single process has part of the cell functioning as an axon and another as a dendrite. They are commonly located within the spinal cord.

It should be noted that there are millions of neurons allotted to the brain. In the past, it was believed that we were all born with a fixed lot of neurons. As we age, these neurons would deplete thereby leading to cognitive decline over time. However, modern research has shown that neuron does regenerate. Yet, what leads to cognitive decline over time, is "gunk" that builds up in the brain. This gunk is the byproduct of the electrochemical processes that happen in the brain and is cleaned up every night when we go to sleep. Therefore, it is vital to get enough sleep. That way, the brain can go about its maintenance process thereby preserving optimal performance.

Chapter 3: The Peripheral Nervous System

At the outset of this book, we focused on the CNS. The CNS is the essential unit that controls the functioning of the entire nervous system. As we have also established, the CNS plays a pivotal role in ensuring that the body is able to sustain life, repair itself and go about daily chores and activities.

At this point, we are going dive into the Peripheral Nervous System (PNS). The PNS is responsible for a myriad of functions and activities. Hence, it is just as important as the CNS, though with a more specialized task.

The PNS is made up of two main components: the somatic nervous system (SNS) and the autonomic nervous system (ANS). Each one of these individual nervous systems provides specific functions to the CNS. As such, they are significant insofar as providing the brain with the information it requires on the movements of the body and essential biological functions.

The Somatic Nervous System

The SNS has a very specific task, that is, to relay information from the limbs to the CNS. The SNS is made up of a network of nervous fibers that allow the brain to control the movement of the limbs. This is what enables walking, sitting, typing, eating, playing sports and so on. Without this network, the brain would be unable to control voluntary movement. Therefore, a person would not be able to move voluntary. Since this is not the case, we can only speculate as to how the body would be controlled.

The SNS controls muscles and their movements through a series of voluntary responses, either stemming from an individual's desire to carry out a specific activity, or as a result of the response which emanates from an external stimulus.

Consider this example:

First, an individual wants to grab an apple. This is a voluntary movement that requires the brain to signal the limbs (arms and hands) to reach out and grab the apple.

Next, the brain receives input from a visual stimulus. The brain has perceived there is a fire. As such, the brain sends a signal to the legs to get moving and hightail away from the fire. In this case, this is a matter of responding to the external stimulus.

Now, it should be noted that the reaction to the fire is part of the ANS, it is worth mentioning that without the SNS, the legs would be unable to make any kind of movement whatsoever. So, the SNS plays a crucial role in survival.

The Autonomic Nervous System

The ANS is incredibly important in the body's sustainment of life. Without it, the essential biological functions, the involuntary kind, would be impossible to carry out. After all, imagine how hard life would be if you have to remember to keep breathing or make a conscious decision to digest food.

As such, the ANS is commonly associated with biological functions that are broken up into two main categories: the sympathetic nervous system and the parasympathetic nervous system.

The Sympathetic Nervous System

The Sympathetic Nervous System is associated with the fight-or-flight response that virtually all living beings have. In humans, this is a response to an external stimulus. In the example of the fire, the reaction to the perceived threat is generated by the Sympathetic Nervous System. This system sends a signal to the CNS which then sends an order to the SNS to get moving.

Also, the Sympathetic Nervous System is considered to be on stand-by and comes into action generally when levels of stress increase. The hormone known as cortisol plays a key role in this situation. When the body detects higher levels of cortisol, the Sympathetic Nervous System kicks into gear.

Here are the main attributes of the sympathetic nervous system:

1. The bronchioles in the lungs are expanded to permit more air into the lungs, which build the oxygenation of the blood and stay aware of the increased blood flow through the lungs as a result of the expanded heart rate.
2. Bladder and sphincter control. This part of the nervous system is associated with bladder and sphincter control at a conscious level. In fact, loss of control of these two functions can be traced back to some kind of damage in this biological function. As a result, care needs to be taken to avoid any potential issues with these functions.
3. The pupils of the eyes become dilated. Since the sympathetic nervous system is regularly enacted when individuals are under stimulation, the dilation of eye pupils is a clear sign of some type of increase in the nervous system's response to the stimulus in question.
4. Increased heart rate. When the heart increases, whether as a result of physical exertion or a stress response, the flow of blood increases thereby leading to greater amounts of oxygen flowing through the body.
5. The digestive system is slowed as a result of the increased response to stress, among other biological functions which are slowed down. This slowdown is the result of the body's need to prioritize resources

with regard to the physiological response that is in course.

6. The adrenal organs epinephrine and norepinephrine. The adrenals are a couple of hormone-creating glands situated over the kidneys that react to stress. Together, the epinephrine and norepinephrine discharged by the adrenal glands have an essential impact on the sympathetic nervous system by increasing heart rate, expanding the bronchioles, and increasing glucose discharge from the liver. Moreover, norepinephrine is likewise known to increase alertness. It might appear to be repetitive that these hormones have indistinguishable activities from the sympathetic neurons, however, hormones have longer enduring impacts than nerve driving forces, so while the underlying battle or flight reaction is interceded by neurons, these hormones serve to fortify and support the reaction.

7. The liver discharges glucose into the circulatory system giving the body an increased caloric supply that will be prepared to control the muscles in the event that it is required.

The Parasympathetic Nervous System

The Parasympathetic Nervous System plays an active role insofar as keeping essential bodily functions moving. As such, the parasympathetic nervous system is commonly called the "feed and breed" system since it controls common procedures that are indispensable for the sustainability of ordinary life. The elements of this system include lowering pulse and heart rate after a spike of the fight-or-flight reaction, regulation of stress hormones such as cortisol and the blood pressure control in addition to biological functions such as breathing, circulation, digestion and sensory management.

Parasympathetic nerves begin in the spine, emerging from the spinal nerves of the central nervous system. The axons of this system are generally very long and stretch out into ganglia throughout the remainder of the body. These ganglia are commonly situated in, or close to, organs, enabling the parasympathetic nervous system to quickly send and receive messages from all over the body. Since the parasympathetic nervous system starts in the spine, it does not ordinarily require conscious thought to activate its functions.

The parasympathetic nervous system begins from average medullary locales (core vague, core tractus solitarius, and dorsal motor core) and is regulated by the nerve center. Vagal efferents reach out from the medulla to postganglionic nerves that innervate the atria by means of ganglia situated in cardiovascular fat cushions with neurotransmission that is adjusted through nicotinic receptors. Postganglionic parasympathetic and sympathetic cholinergic nerves at that point influence heart muscarinic receptors.

Parasympathetic enactment can influence atrioventricular nodal conduction intervened prevalently through the left vagus nerve. Besides, muscarinic receptors on vein dividers can cause vasorelaxation through nitric oxide (NO), regulated pathway however can likewise cause vasoconstriction by legitimately enacting smooth muscle. Subsequently, in spite of the fact that the sympathetic nervous system affects cardiovascular physiology in an all-or-none kind of reaction, the parasympathetic nervous system can have a specific balance at different levels.

Vagus nerve afferent actuation, beginning incidentally, can adjust efferent sympathetic and parasympathetic capacity centrally and at the degree of the baroreceptor.

Efferent vagal nerve actuation can have tonic and basal impacts that hinder the sympathetic initiation and arrival of norepinephrine at the presynaptic level. Acetylcholine discharge from parasympathetic nerve terminals will initiate ganglionic nicotinic receptors that thusly enact muscarinic receptors at the cell level. Cardiovascular impacts incorporate pulse decrease by the hindrance of the sympathetic nervous system and by direct hyperpolarization of sinus nodal cells.

Chapter 4: Stress and the Nervous System

Stress is undoubtedly one of the most widely discussed topics in modern society. The hustle and bustle of everyday life make it hard for us to get a grip on our feelings and the environment around us.

The fact of the matter is that no matter how many coping strategies we may have, stress will eventually catch up to us. Furthermore, tolerance to stress varies greatly from person to person. For some folks, stress is a part of daily life. As such, they are more accustomed to dealing with prolonged periods of stress. In contrast, others may feel more overwhelmed especially when stress moments spike at any given point.

For all of the negative press that stress receives, the truth is that stress is a very useful response as it is an evolutionary trait that humans developed over time. The reason why stress exists is to help ensure survival. Plain and simple.

If we go back to the early days of humanity, early humans had to contend with the elements, large predatory animals and an endless shortage of food and water. That is why stress emerged as a response to external stimuli. The human body needed some type of signal to alert the individual that something wasn't right, and action needed to be taken.

For instance, is a human encountered a bear, such an encounter would hardly be pleasant. In fact, the bear might feel threatened and its fight or flight mechanism would spur it to attack. Such an encounter could lead to loss of life on the human's part, or in the best of cases, a very good run while attempting to get away from the bear.

This example underscores the function of stress as part of the human condition. As humans began improving agricultural techniques and the domestication of animals, hunter-gatherer civilizations gave way to agricultural-based ones. Then, as civilization flourished in various parts of the world, the need to engage other large predators diminished. Fast forward to our time, and the need to engage the fight or flight mechanism is limited to instances of potential harm such as a robbery, physical violence and so on.

So, human civilization has moved away from those elements which induced the evolution of stress, yet the stress remains hardwired in the human body. Perhaps we might go through another evolution in which the stress response becomes more attuned to a less stressful environment. In the meantime, we have the nervous system that we inherited from our ancestors.

Stress hormones

Stress hormones are unleashed when a perceived threat is processed by the brain. The brain then signals the body to begin production of several hormones. One of the most common hormones is adrenaline.

Adrenaline is a hormone which kicks the body into high gear. It stimulates the response from the immune system, locks down the digestive tract and improves blood circulation and airflow to the brain. This is the rush that most people get when they practice extreme sports and other types of dangerous activities. It is also the same rush that a person gets when they feel their life might be in danger.

Another hormone that plays a key role in stress is called cortisol. This hormone isn't normally produced by the body unless there is a stress response to some kind of stimulus. Cortisol signals the body to hoard energy and enter "survival mode". In fact, when a person engages in a crash diet in which they drastically reduce the caloric intake in a short period of time, the body may begin to emit cortisol as a stress signal, an SOS if you will, and thereby force the metabolism to go on lockdown. This means that the individual plateaus in their diet and no matter how long they stay on it, they lose weight.

Burnout

When a person is exposed to prolonged periods of stress, such as months or even years, a condition known as "burnout" may take place. Burnout is a condition in which the nervous system becomes so overloaded by stress that it simply begins to shutdown as a means of protecting the body.

In this condition, the individual may begin to feel chronic fatigue, pain, and constant illness. The nervous system may become permanently damaged leading to irregular sleep, digestive and metabolic disorders in addition hypersensitivity to stress. One associated condition to prolonged stress is insulin resistance which is a common marker for diabetes.

Burnout may also result from a single event in which the nervous system becomes completely overwhelmed. Think of a traffic accident, a violent incident or perhaps the loss of a loved one. In this circumstance, Post-Traumatic Stress Disorder (PTSD) may ensue thus leaving the individual with "frayed nerves".

In olden times, frayed nerves were equated to a "nervous breakdown". A nervous breakdown in an incident in which a person has been exposed to stress, usually intense stress over a short period of time, thereby leaving the individual exhausted and in need of recovery. Think of an individual working long hours, over a period of several weeks in order to get a project done. This intense regimen will leave the person in need of recovery from such an event, but without the long-term effects that may emerge as a result of months or even years of prolonged stress.

Recovering from stress

Recovering from stress may be a combination of nutrition and medication. For folks who are under intense periods of stress, such as suffering from PTSD, antidepressants may be prescribed. In other cases, some type of psychotherapy may be recommended.

The fact of the matter is that recovery from stress may necessitate complete isolation from the source of stress. Furthermore, the individual may need extended periods of rest, sleep and recreation in order to level out hormone production. Ultimately, the individual can make a full recovery from the effect of stress, but it may require a complete lifestyle overhaul especially when the individual has been immersed in a violent and/or abusive environment.

If you, or a loved one, are going through a prolonged period of stress, it is best to consult your physician about the treatment options available to you. It is best to address this issue sooner rather than later. That way, you can avoid the development of potentially serious long-term effects.

PART II: THE VAGUS NERVE

Chapter 5: The Vagus Nerve

After discussing the nervous system and its components, we will now focus on one of the most interesting elements that comprise the nervous system: the vagus nerve.

If you haven't heard about this nerve before, don't worry. While its existence has been known for some time, doctors and researchers didn't really understand it until recently. Modern research conducted on this nerve has led to many interesting discoveries.

So, what is the vagus nerve?

The name "vagus" is Latin for "wanderer". This means that the vagus nerve wanders and meanders throughout the body. It is a cranial nerve that runs throughout the entire body. It is associated to the parasympathetic nervous system (PNS). As such, it is the main highway by which the Central Nervous System (CNS) communicates with the PNS. As such, it is tremendously important in regulating all of the essential bodily functions that the PNS regulates.

Given the fact that it is so important, it is surprising just how overlooked this nerve actually is. That is why this section is dedicated to understanding what it is and what it does. In addition, we will be discussing how your understanding of this nerve can help you increase your overall health and wellness. So, sit tight because we are going to be discussing quite a bit of information here. You will surely find this to be insightful as well as fascinating.

We will begin by looking deep into two crucial components of the vagus nerve, the Pneumogastric Nerve and the Ventral Branch of the vagus nerve.

The Pneumogastric Nerve

Before modern research on the vagus nerve was conducted, the name it commonly received was the "pneumogastric nerve". It had earned this designation since the vagus nerve is responsible for the regulation of the heart, lungs and digestive tract.

As the pneumogastric nerve is responsible for ensuring the proper functioning of these systems through the PNS. The PNS relies on the pneumogastric nerve to relay the right information to and from the CNS and the brain. Yet, the fact that the pneumogastric nerve starts in the brain and works its way down into the lungs, heart and digestive tract, it essentially becomes one of the most important neural networks in the body. Needless to say, that if something goes haywire in the pneumogastric nerve, it can lead to serious consequences in the rest of the body.

The pneumogastric nerve begins in the brain and leaves through the medulla oblongata. Then, it basically runs straight through the middle of the body down the neck, chest and into the abdomen. The pneumogastric nerve has ramifications, or branches, that touch upon the main organ systems described earlier.

First, the pneumogastric nerve connects into the laryngeal nerve and then curves around the subclavian artery so that it emerges between the trachea and the esophagus. This is where it is able to regulate the functioning of the lungs. As such, this nerve enables the PNS to regulate breathing.

Next, the nerve runs down from the subclavian artery into the superior vena cava. From there, it moves on onto the bronchus before settling into the vagal trunk that passes through the diaphragm. It also connects into the carotid artery in which then allows it to link with the cardiac tissue.

This is the point at which the pneumogastric nerve enables the PNS to hook up with the heart.

As the pneumogastric nerve makes its way down the esophagus and through the diaphragm, it is now able to link up with the digestive tract. This is what permits the PNS to regulate digestion.

As you can see, the pneumogastric nerve is truly an intricate piece of hardware which enables the PNS to regulate some of the most complex bodily functions. Needless to say, the body would not be able to function adequately without the pneumogastric nerve.

The pneumogastric nerve has the following branches which serve as means of communication among the entire routing of this nerve:

- Anterior vagal trunk
- Branches to the esophageal plexus
- Branches to the pulmonary plexus
- Hering-Breuer reflex in alveoli
- Inferior cervical cardiac branch
- Pharyngeal nerve
- Posterior vagal trunk
- Recurrent laryngeal nerve
- Superior cervical cardiac branches of vagus nerve
- Superior laryngeal nerve
- Thoracic cardiac branches

These branches are what enables the pneumogastric job to do its job effectively. When the system is firing on all cylinders, the communication flows effortlessly and regulation happens without a hitch. However, when there is a disruption in communication, or if the pneumogastric nerve becomes altered in any fashion, disruptions may occur leading to any number of potential medical conditions. Later on, we will dig deeper into these conditions.

The Ventral Branch of the Vagus Nerve

The emergence of Polyvagal Theory has allowed for a deeper understanding of the nervous system and its effects on the overall wellbeing of the body. Generally speaking, the vagus nerve is considered as one mega-unit which regulates a number of vital biological systems. We have covered this in-depth throughout the book.

At this point, we can dive straight into the discussion of Porges' Polyvagal approach explains the effect of the vagus nerve on the body. Since the vagus nerve is at the forefront of the PNS, it has a calming effect on the SNS.

Let's elaborate on that point further.

For instance, a person has been involved in a minor car accident, a fender-bender if you will. The incident itself is rather stressful though it does not bear any major consequences. As such, the individual is just shaken up and in need of some rest in order to get over what has occurred. In this example, the SNS kicked into high gear at the occurrence of the accident since the brain perceived a potential threat, that being the car accident. After closer inspection, there were no injuries, and everything proved to be rather innocuous.

If the PNS did not exist, there would be no way for the SNS to essentially shut off; the individual would remain at a constant state of stress and anxiety. Needless to say, they would not be able to sleep or eat due to the stress on them. This harkens back to the point we made earlier about prolonged stress and the effect it has on the overall nervous system.

After the brain has perceived that the threat is over, the PNS takes over and begins to bring back bodily functions down to normal parameters. This means that pulse and heart rate return to normal, blood pressure decreases, and the metabolism resumes normal operations. In the theory, all is well, and the individual makes a full recovery after a good night's sleep.

As a corollary, it is important to highlight the fact that sleep is a great equalizer. This is why you tend to feel sleepy after a significant spike in stress. Sleep allows the PNS to regulate body functions and bring the entire system back to normal. If you are unable to sleep, then the lasting effects will take much longer to become subdued thereby leading you to feel as if you had been hit by a train.

Based on the previous example, the ANS was seen as a mix of both active and passive roles. Of course, the active part only springs into action when there is the need for it, while the passive role hums along in the background.

That being said, the Polyvagal theory suggests that there is a third component of the system. A component which Porges called the "social engagement" system. In a way, this is a smart system that requires the removal of any perceived threat. What this implies is that we need to be able to discern when there is a threat and when there is not. When this discrimination occurs, it is not the "passive" side that takes over, but rather, it is the social engagement side of the equation.

So, how do these three systems work in tandem?

The SNS kicks into gear when there is a threat. Everything goes into high gear. The threat subsides and the brain determines the threat is over. Then, the social engagement system kicks in and alerts the SNS giving it the "all clear" signal. As such, the only thing that the SNS does is regulate the parameters of bodily functions; the SNS and the social engagement system work in an on/off basis. It should be noted that the default setting for the body is the activation of the social engagement system. The SNS is meant to be used only in case of emergency.

The ventral branch comes into play when the social engagement system is in control. The ventral branch essentially regulates everything that happens above the diaphragm in such a manner that the body is able to continuously regulate its responses.

In other words, the brain perceives a potential threat but then quickly discards it. The social engagement system clicks off and clicks back on almost instantly.

How does such a thing work?

For example, you are walking down the street at night and a person approaches. You are concerned that this may be a stranger who means harm. As you get closer, you realize it is a friendly neighbor. The warning issued by the brain did not last long enough for the social engagement system to be shut off and the SNS activated. However, the brain did issue a warning with alerted the social engagement system to be on standby. If the warning was real, then the SNS would kick in and the appropriate response would ensue.

According to this example based on the Polyvagal theory, the social engagement system is the default system for the human body. Consequently, this brings to light the fact that the SNS is only meant to be active for very brief periods of time. As a result, we can infer that prolonged periods of SNS activation can lead to a serious drain on the body's overall energy and wellbeing. Hence, it is vitally important to help the body calm down.

As we will discuss later on, this calming, or soothing effect can be achieved through the right stimulation of the vagal nerve. Moreover, it is helpful to look at this stimulation at a broader level insofar as the calming and soothing of the entire nervous system thereby leading the body to achieve proper balance among all of its functions.

One other important consideration to take into account is that prolonged stress on the nervous system can lead to some of the disorders which we will discuss in an upcoming chapter. That is why we would like to point out the importance of calming the nervous system throughout this book. That way you can begin to see immediate results. In fact, just by being able to take some time away from the main sources of stress in your life, you will be able to see a quick turnaround in the way you feel and the way your body reacts to the various stimuli around you. Of course, we will delve deep into this topic in due time.

In the meantime, it is highly recommended that you make an assessment of the various aspects that may be causing you to feel stressed out. Sure, there may be a stressor which you have little control over. For example, you may have very little control over your job. Still, you have control over the ways in which you can dissipate that negative energy that may be overloading your nervous system, in particular, the SNS thereby leading you to walk around with an overloaded PNS.

Chapter 6: Functions of the Vagus Nerve

In earlier chapters, we have mentioned the main function of the vagus nerve. As such, we have pointed out the importance of the vagus nerve and its pivotal role in keeping the entire body's biological system humming along.

In this chapter, we are going to focus on the specific functions of the vagus nerve and highlight the points in which the vagus nerve may be vulnerable. Thus, we would like to further underscore the importance of taking proper care of the nervous system thereby ensuring proper functioning of the vagus nerve and associated biological systems.

Main functions of the vagus nerve

The vagus nerve is one large highway that conducts the flow of information from the biological systems that it controls up to the CNS. This is the main raison d'etre of the vagus nerve. In a manner of speaking, the vagus nerve is like a central command post in which the information comes and goes. Consequently, the vagus nerve provides the CNS with all of the data it needs to keep the body alive.

Let's assume that the vagus nerve simply stops working for whatever reason. In such a situation, the person would simply die. How so? If the vagus nerve stops sending information to the CNS, the CNS may conclude that the heart and lungs have stopped functioning. Therefore, the brain may have no choice but to begin shutting down other organ systems as well. This type of response may lead doctors to place a patient on life support.

This example highlights the importance that the vagus nerve has on the body's overall ability to sustain life. Now, let's assume that the vagus nerve is functioning properly, but there is some kind of damage to one of the organ systems. In that case, the vagus nerve relays the data on the damage to the organ system back up to the CNS. The brain then sends back the information through the vagus nerve and adjusts accordingly. For instance, if one lung is severely damaged, the brain may choose to shut down that lung and shift all of the breathing functions to the other healthy lung. This is enough to keep the body alive though not necessarily at peak performance.

In addition, the vagus nerve is the main command post for the digestive system. This is a crucial function to consider since the digestive system provides the body with the nutrition it needs to repair itself, fuel movement and keep cells running along. Hence, the digestive system needs close attention. This causal link between the digestive system and the CNS explains why folks who have undergone a traumatic experience often experience digestive distress. When the nervous system suffers a significant jolt, it is not uncommon to see that it has serious repercussions on the entire network controlled by the vagus nerve.

So, let's move on and take a deeper look at the specific functions that are associated with the vagus nerve.

The Visceral Somatic Function

Given the fact that the vagus nerve is part of the Autonomic Nervous System (ANS), it is inextricably linked to the entire body. Think of it as a main highway that receives traffic from all over the region even if the majority of motorists don't actually plan to stay in that particular area. In a way, the main traffic is just passing through.

Based on that premise, any disruption in the flow of traffic in that area may lead to disruption in the flow of traffic in other seemingly unrelated areas. The same goes for the nervous system and biological functions.

When we refer to a somatic function, we are talking about the reaction that comes as a result of the stimuli in the environment surrounding an organism. In this case, the human body is the organism immersed in a given environment. We have also discussed ad nauseum how the body reacts to stimuli by enacting the SNS at the sight of a perceived threat.

As such, the somatic function that the vagus nerve plays is one of constant monitoring and regulation. Think of it as one large pressure valve that looks to regulate the build-up within a large engine. If too much pressure builds up, then the engine may explode. The same goes for the nervous system.

With that in mind, there is one interesting bit of good news... if we could call it that. The body is adept at adjusting to its environment. So, if the individual finds themselves consistently inundated by stressful situations, there is the possibility that the body will become adjusted to such levels of stress. In a way, it creates a "new normal".

An example of this attitude can be seen in the so-called "adrenaline junkies". These people become addicted to extreme sports due to the exhilaration that they get from engaging in a dangerous activity. However, they consistently need to up the ante since their nervous system constantly adjusts to the level of danger in each activity. So, in order to get the same rush, they need to overload their nervous system more and more. Otherwise, they may not find the same amount of enjoyment in the same activities.

As far as the visceral function is concerned, the vagus nerve is constantly tracking the performance of the body's internal organ systems. As a matter of fact, it is designed with a number of automatic switches that are intended to protect the body from grievous damage. Think of these switches like circuit breakers in an electrical system. When the system is overloaded by the electrical current, the circuit breaker is tripped thereby protecting the entire system. If no such breaker existed, the wiring would overheat potentially causing a fire.

The vagus nerve has built-in parameters that prevent the body from overexerting itself to the point where permanent damage is done to organs. Consider this situation:

A person who has been working non-stop for a week may find that after going on little to no sleep, they simply crash and sleep for an extended period of time. This reaction is triggered in the nervous system in order to prevent the heart from literally burning out. This is why drug consumption, the kind that disrupts the nervous system, making it prone for individuals to suffer from cardiac arrest. Since the substance wreaks havoc with the PNS natural regulation mechanisms, the body keeps going until it eventually shuts down.

A good example of this can be seen in modern cars. The car's computer shuts the engine down when it diagnoses a potentially serious problem in the engine. The car's control computer module shuts off the flow of gas, for example, in order to keep the engine from completely failing. The car will restart once the issue has been corrected.

So, just like a car's control module, the vagus nerve serves as the body's main regulation unit. This protects the body's vital organs from failing altogether at which point death would ensue. This is why optimal performance from the vagus nerve is essential to ensuring the body's overall optimal performance.

The Physical Motor Function

Since the vagus nerve is part of the overall ANS, it is also connected to the body's peripheral nervous system which controls the movement of limbs. As such, the vagus nerve is involved in the motor functions of the body.

Now, the vagus nerve itself does not regulate movement, but it does regulate the biological functions that aid movement. The following example will illustrate this point.

When a person engages in physical activity, the CNS broadcasts the necessary signals to the limbs for movement, be it running, swimming, and so on. However, the heart is also responsible for supply blood to the muscles while the lungs need to provide oxygen. Furthermore, there is an increased metabolic response as the body needs to create the energy it requires to sustain the level of physical activity. If the activity exceeds the heart's capacity to pump blood and the lungs' ability to provide oxygen, then the individual may simply get tired and stop moving.

This example highlights how important the vagus nerve is when taking movement into account. High-performance athletes have trained not only for their sport, but also develop stamina. Now, you may have heard of this term, yet it is generally associated to endurance, that is, sustaining physical activity over longer periods of time. But the fact of the matter is that stamina is the body's ability to provide the elements the body needs to sustain prolonged periods of physical activity.

Consequently, the vagus nerve is able to recognize these increased levels of physical activity and make the necessary adjustments so that muscles get the elements they need in order to keep going. It should be noted that the vagus nerve will also recognize when an athlete is becoming overexerted. At which point, the athlete may feel like they can't go on anymore. This is the body's protective measures that keep it from causing serious damage.

This last point illustrates the importance of keeping a balanced nervous system so that the vagus nerve can perform its functions appropriately thereby allowing the body's organ systems to provide the elements that the body requires.

Essential biological functions

At this point, we have widely discussed the essential biological functions that the vagus nerve regulates. These functions are what basically keeps the body alive. After all, if your heart stops breathing, then chances are you are not going to make it.

With that in mind, it is important to note that when the vagus nerve is not functioning at 100%, that is, when there is some kind of disruption, the essential biological systems may begin to go haywire. In some cases, it might be a slow and progressive disruption while in other cases it may be a sudden and shocking disruption.

Let's consider two possible scenarios:

An individual who has been working a stressful job begins to feel the effects of chronic stress over months or even years of accumulated stress. Suddenly, they may develop cardiac conditions, anxiety or even chronic digestive disorders. Yet, the progression of these conditions was so subtle that the person didn't really feel much of a difference.

On the flip side, there is a person who underwent a major traumatic incident, for instance, the loss of a loved one. The stress caused by the sudden loss of a dear person may cause a sudden overload to the nervous system. This sudden overload may lead to the onset of any of the aforementioned conditions. This may prompt swift intervention by medical professionals in order to address the onset of the symptoms the person is experiencing.

In either case, the vagus nerve can come under attack. At this point, there is s serious need for treatment which can correct the imbalances in the nervous system thus promoting recovery from the overwhelming effects on the nervous system. Given these considerations, the following chapter will go into great detail about the conditions that are beset by disruptions in the vagus nerve's proper functioning. In fact, you may be surprised that some of the most common conditions that you may be familiar with can be addressed by balancing out the vagus nerve's functions.

Chapter 7: Dysfunctions of the Vagus Nerve

Thus far, we have focused heavily on the functions of the vagus nerve and what it is intended to do. However, we have only briefly touched upon the various consequences of a dysfunctional vagus nerve.

The vagus nerve, on its own, does not break down or show signs of dysfunction on its own. Barring some sort of physiological issue in which a person is born with a dysfunctional vagus nerve, the dysfunctions that may occur to it are generally the result of the strain the nervous system is put under. This is important to note as the nervous system is designed to take its share of wear and tear. Nevertheless, even something as strong and robust as the nervous system can, and will, eventually begin to break down.

Unless the individual is faced with a sudden shock, say an accident, in which the vagus nerve is severely damaged, the dysfunctions of the vagus nerve occur after a prolonged period of strain. Therefore, the wear and tear that the vagus nerve suffers is a progressive condition. In fact, it can be so subtle, that a person may not know that something is wrong until it is too late. For example, a person may not be fully aware of the stress he has in his body, until he has a heart attack. At this point, doctors may discover that there is something wrong with the person's nervous system. By that point, the results may be irreversible.

This is why we can infer that, barring physiological causes, the vagus nerve becomes damaged as a result of prolonged periods of stress and overwhelming strain on the nervous system. As such, it is important to address nervous system health at once. In a later chapter, we will focus on specific means of stimulating the vagus nerve. Nevertheless, it is worth mentioning that adequate rest, sleep and proper nutrition are the core tenets of building a healthy nervous system. In doing so, you will get a leg up on recovery from any of the conditions that we will mention in this chapter.

So, let's take a closer look at the various conditions that may be onset by dysfunctions of the vagus nerve.

Anxiety

Anxiety is a condition that affects people from all walks of life. It affects men and women alike, while it affects children, teens, and adults just the same. The root cause of anxiety is stress. As such, it is important to determine the sources of that stress.

Stressors abound in the world around us. These can range from purely emotional causes to physiological causes. That is why we are going to explore both angles. That way, we can gain a broader perspective on anxiety and its relation to the vagus nerve.

As we have mentioned throughout this book, the vagus nerve is part of the PNS. The PNS is charged with the task of bringing the body's bodily functions back to within acceptable parameters. When the nervous system is maxed out, the PNS may have trouble regulating the body back to normal parameters.

Consider this situation:

A person who is consistently under stress due to a violent environment in which he lives. This could be a country at war, a rough neighborhood, or a break down in the law and order of a place. The person is constantly fearing for his safety and that of his loved ones. Such people are constantly worried about attacks, gunfire or any other type of violent attack. Since the fight or flight response is active all the time, there will come a time with the PNS will be unable to regulate the nervous system. Eventually, the vagus nerve begins to suffer the effect of this overload. So, once the person is finally removed from this violent environment, he may be unable to return to normal. He may suffer from chronic anxiety and require medication in order to help him get back to normal.

There is an individual who recently lost his job. While he had a comfortable financial position, now he feels at a loss. He feels like his skills and talents have not been appreciated. This state of loss leads to overloading the nervous system. Since the person is unable to get over the loss of his job, he can't seem to get any peace. In the end, the vagus nerve begins to pay the price since the individual cannot get back on track. In the end, a condition of chronic anxiety may ensure especially since it doesn't seem to be any respite from the feelings produced by this event.

Both of these events, although somewhat extreme, serve to show how the PNS eventually becomes overwhelmed and unable to regulate the body back to its normal parameters. As such, the anxious state becomes the "new normal" for the body. At this point, the individual may have no choice but to go on medication. Nevertheless, addressing the damage done to the vagus nerve may very well be enough to sort out the issue and help the individual get back on track.

Depression

Depression is usually associated to anxiety though depression is not necessarily the consequence of anxiety. In fact, a person may suffer from both depression and anxiety given the circumstances they are forced to endure. Under this consideration, depression can be differentiated from anxiety insofar as depression is a constant state of sadness and gloom. The individual suffering from depression may feel there is nothing to live for. If unattended, depression can lead to thoughts of harming oneself. In the worst of cases, depression may lead to suicide.

Just like anxiety, the causes for depression may vary from a purely physiological one, such as irregular brain chemistry, to purely psychological ones such as feelings of profound sadness as a result of the loss of loved one, significant life changes and even untreated anxiety. In such cases, depression may reach a point in which psychotherapy and medication may be insufficient to help an individual return to normalcy. In fact, some folks may require hospitalization in a proper mental care facility especially when they have shown signs of harming themselves.

The onset of depression generally has its origins in an overloaded nervous system. When the individual is not removed from the environment which is causing them significant stress, they may end up suffering from physical effects such as chronic fatigue, low immune response, or even impaired cognitive ability. All of these physical conditions can be traced back to poor regulation from the vagus nerve.

Hence, the need for proper regulation from the vagus nerve will ensure that the nervous system has the opportunity to recover from the stressful events that caused it to become overloaded in the first place. However, this is a personal decision that every individual needs to make. It might seem like a no-brainer, that is to extricate oneself from a stressful environment, but the fact of the matter is that it may not always be possible to do so.

Depression is generally treated with a combination of medication and psychotherapy. But the fact is that medication only helps to manage the symptoms but does very little to address the root cause of the depression itself. This is what psychotherapy is for. Yet, the process of therapy may be even more stressful as the patient is asked to confront the stressful events causing depression. For instance, if the depression can be traced back to a traumatic event in childhood, the patient may have a major episode when asked to relive this event.

While both medication and therapy are viable means of dealing with depression, doctors often look at the importance of treating the vagus nerve. When this vagus nerve is addressed, many of the symptoms of depression begin to subside. For example, mindfulness and meditation have been known to help depression sufferers. Now, meditation in itself is not the solution. The apparent solution lies in the fact that meditation has a soothing effect on the nervous system. Thus, it is this soothing effect that helps the vagus nerve return to normal operations.

Panic attacks

Another condition associated with vagus nerve dysfunction is known as panic attacks. Panic attacks allude to repetitive, sudden episodes that include unpleasant physical, intellectual manifestations, and social signs. These episodes involve anxiety rising to the level in which the individual is unable to cope with the overwhelming emotions that overcome them. As a result, they may feel completely inundated with worry and stress that goes beyond any coping mechanism they may employ.

The following signs are indicative of a panic attack:

- Significant conduct changes identified with the attacks (for instance, evading activity or spots due to being paranoid about having a panic attack).
- Consistent worry about having another panic assault or the outcomes of a panic assault (for example, having a heart attack).
- A panic attack is an unexpected inclination of serious dread or distress that spikes in a matter of minutes. It incorporates distressing physical and psychological manifestations just like behavioral signs.

- Panic disorder alludes to repetitive, unforeseen panic attacks (e.g., heart palpitations, perspiring, trembling) trailed by in any event one month.

Specific physical symptoms may include:

- Feelings of warmth or cold
- Chest torment or uneasiness
- Dizziness and lightheadedness
- Gag reflex
- Increased heart rate
- Perspiration
- Feelings of loneliness and isolation
- Shortness of breath
- Trembling or shaking

These symptoms fuel a negative feedback loop in which the individual feels terrible to be with, and the addition of these symptoms only makes the individual feel worse thereby fueling the attack to even greater depths. As a result, the onset of a panic attack is enough to keep the sufferer in a constant state of anxiety.

Much like depression and anxiety, panic attacks can be treated with a combination of medication and therapy. Generally speaking, this course of treatment is effective although it should be noted that treatment alleviates the symptoms that lead to the onset of a panic attack but not the root cause itself. Medication is quite adept at helping regulate brain chemistry but does little to aid the nervous system in regulating essential functions such as those related to the PNS. As a result, feelings and symptoms subside but little is actually done to promote the health of the individual sufferer in the long run.

Furthermore, conventional treatments don't do very much in terms of helping the vagus nerve recover to its full capacity. So, even if the individual strives to make a full recovery, the fact that the vagus nerve tends to be overlooked makes a full recovery rather complicated. As such, it is important that treatment also is centered on helping the vagus nerve bounce back to its normal state.

Inflammation and Autoimmune diseases

Inflammation is a condition in which tissue swells up in an attempt to isolate an area that is affected by some sort of aggressor. One of the most common areas of inflammation is the digestive system. Inflammation of the digestive system is common as a result of food allergies or overconsumption of certain types of foods.

Nevertheless, inflammation can happen in any part of the body. This also affects the nervous system as it is quite possible for the CNS to experience inflammation as a result of excessive periods of stress. Swelling in the brain may occur, not just as a consequence of a severe blow to the head, but also of prolonged periods of sleep deprivation, substance abuse (drugs, alcohol, caffeine, painkillers, and so on) and high levels of stress.

When the nervous system becomes overwhelmed, the brain sends a distress signal to the immune system to begin a lockdown on the afflicted parts of the body. However, inflammation in the nervous system is nothing compared to inflammation in a local part of the body. For instance, if you fall and sprain your ankle, the body uses inflammation to protect the sprained ankle.

In the case of the nervous system, we are talking about a significant amount of the body that is affected. Furthermore, the nervous system runs the entire body. Consequently, inflammation of the nervous system means inflammation throughout the entire body. Needless to say, this can lead to all sorts of conditions ranging from mild pain and discomfort to serious conditions which may end up becoming chronic.

When the nervous system is out of whack, the immune system, the body's line of defense against illness, also goes out of whack. When the immune system is not fully online, a recurring illness may set in. But beyond getting constantly sick, the immune system may trigger what is known as an "autoimmune disease".

Autoimmune diseases, by definition, are when the immune system believes that a healthy part of the body is somehow causing the body harm. So, it attacks the body causing damage to an area that it's supposed to protect. If that sounds contradictory, it really is.

The nature of autoimmune diseases is not quite understood by modern medical science. There is any number of causes for such ailments. But almost all of them can be traced back to some sort of issue within the nervous system. Again, unless there is some underlying physiological or genetic factor causing the illness, autoimmune afflictions are almost always caused by dysfunctions in the nervous system.

Examples of such illnesses include Lupus, Psoriasis, Sjogren's Syndrome, Rheumatoid Arthritis and Irritable Bowel Syndrome, among others. Autoimmune diseases lead to degenerative conditions that are almost always irreversible. One such example is the kidney damage that Lupus causes its sufferers. Lupus attacks healthy tissue in the kidneys to the extent of rendering them useless. The ultimate consequence is chronic renal failure. Transplant in Lupus patients is highly risky as the immune system not only tends to reject the new organ but may also require the patient to be on lifelong immunosuppressor treatment. Thus, autoimmune diseases are certainly to be taken seriously.

Chronic conditions – Fibromyalgia

One of the points we have made about dysfunctions of the vagus nerve is the emergence of chronic conditions. By chronic, we understand that these are conditions that are not going away any time soon. In fact, chronic conditions are generally ailments which the person must live with for the rest of their lives. Needless to say, this is not a fun situation to be in.

One of the most common chronic conditions that develop as a result of dysfunctions in the vagus nerve is Fibromyalgia. Fibromyalgia is a disorder described as widespread musculoskeletal torment highlighted by weakness, pain, memory issues, and psychological distress. Specialists accept that Fibromyalgia amplifies difficult sensations by influencing the manner in which the brain processes pain.

Side effects now and again start after a physical injury, medical procedure, contamination or significant mental pressure. In different cases, side effects progressively build up after some time with no single trigger activating an onset of the condition.

While there is no remedy for fibromyalgia, an assortment of prescriptions can help control manifestations. Exercise, unwinding and stress-decrease measures likewise may help. This underscores the need that the vagus nerve requires.

Indications of Fibromyalgia include:

- **Exhaustion**. Individuals with Fibromyalgia regularly feel drained, despite the fact that they report getting regular sleep. Rest is regularly disturbed by agony, and numerous patients with fibromyalgia have other disruptions, for example, fretful legs or even sleep apnea.

- **Far-reaching discomfort**. The unpleasantness related to Fibromyalgia frequently is depicted as a consistent dull pain that has gone on for three months or more. To be viewed as far-reaching, the discomfort must happen on both sides of the body and specifically underneath in the lower body such as the legs.

- **Mental distress**. A side effect generally alluded to as "fibro-mist" which weakens the capacity to concentrate, focus and conduct mental tasks.

Fibromyalgia frequently exists together with other uncomfortable conditions, such as:

- Interstitial cystitis or unpleasant bladder discomfort
- Temporomandibular joint disorders
- Headache leading to possible migraines

As per the definition of chronic conditions, chronic pain doesn't go away on its own. In fact, the individual may experience such conditions for months or even years. Painkillers only mask the symptoms while hardly addressing the actual root cause of the ailment. This is why a closer look at the nervous system may reveal the potential root cause and pathway to relief.

Additionally, vagus nerve dysfunctions manifest themselves throughout the body. So, if a person is suffering from Fibromyalgia, they may not just experience pain the lower extremities but may experience this situation in their hands and arms. For instance, sufferers of this condition often complain of numbness in their hands. This is especially disconcerting when the individual is unable to complete tasks they usually would. As a result, the ailment only fuels the negative feedback loop that is created by the chronic condition itself.

Headaches and migraines

When most individuals hear the term "headache" they regularly think about an extreme headache. What they cannot deny is that headache is a neurological sickness and that there are various different subtypes of headache. Get some answers concerning the different sorts of headache underneath.

Given the fact that it is neurological in nature, it is related to the nervous system in one way or another. Headaches that are not related to stress, such as after a long day at work or school, can be traced back to some sort of nervous system dysfunction. Now, it is entirely possible that headaches can be caused by physical injury such as a concussion sustained in an accident. But beyond clearly identifiable physiological causes, there is little room to doubt that headaches have an origin in neurological causes.

Generally speaking, headaches are discomfort and pain located in the cranial region. In other cases, headaches may extend to the neck and even shoulders. In other cases, a headache may be located in one specific part of the head while in other cases it may simply be a blanket pain that covers the entire head. Regardless of the nature and location of the pain, the main thing to keep in mind is that it is there to being with.

Migraines are generally distinguishable from regular headaches in that they have specific triggers. These triggers may vary from being in crowded places to hearing certain types of sounds. Others may experience migraines when they find themselves inside a movie theater in the midst of a loud action sequence.

Migraines are generally described as stronger than usual headaches that may be accompanied by blurry vision, sensitivity to light and/or sound, nausea, and even digestive distress. For some folks, migraines can be so debilitating that they cannot think properly and are unable to visually focus on any object. This makes tasks such as driving virtually impossible.

Prolonged exposure to stress is also another common source of headaches and migraines. When a person is subject to long hours, little rest and sleep deprivation, headaches may become chronic. It should be noted that the headache itself is not caused by the stress that is being experienced; it is caused by the overload the nervous system is underway. In that case, the vagus nerve's inability to properly regulate the PNS may lead to the sufferer being unable to control the triggers that set off headaches. As such, a chronic condition may be diagnosed if the individual finds themselves suffering from headaches at least 3 days a week, or 14 days out of a month. In the worst of cases, a sufferer may find themselves going consecutive days with headaches. In such situations, medication is almost always the only course of treatment.

Alternative forms of treatment for headaches include meditation and relaxation. This treatment is considered successful since it is aimed at helping the nervous system calm down and help the PNS regulate bodily functions back to normal.

Breathing conditions

Considering that the vagus nerve controls the lungs and heart, it is safe to assume that any dysfunctions in the vagus nerve may lead to breathing issues. In short, breathing issues as a result of the vagus nerve being out of whack can be seen in improper breathing. What this implies is that the body cannot produce enough oxygen for the entire body's functions. When this occurs, the blood cannot carry enough oxygen to the brain and other parts of the body. The end result may be poor cognitive skills and inadequate cell regeneration. If this should be the case, then the suffering may not be able to recuperate well illness and have difficulty sleeping.

Symptoms of poor breathing include:

- Shallow breathing
- Shortness of breath
- Constant labored breathing
- Poor stamina when engaging in physical activity
- Improper circulation
- Lightheadedness and dizziness

While this list is not exhaustive, it serves to prove that poor breathing can be truly disruptive in a person's day to day routine. Moreover, inadequate breathing can lead to long-term cognitive impairment as the brain cannot function properly on low levels of oxygen. Consequently, it is necessary for the brain to be fully oxygenated.

The vagus nerve must then be repaired in order to ensure that proper oxygen absorption takes place. In addition, when the vagus nerve is out of balance, it can lead to cardiac issues solely based on the lack of oxygen in the blood. As such, it is important to pay close attention to breathing.

Long-term pulmonary damage may also ensue as a result of improper breathing. The lungs may be forced to work overtime in order to extract as much oxygen as possible from the air that it receives. Consequently, this may place undue stress on the lungs. If the person happens to live in a place with poor air quality, this may also lead to other degenerative conditions. So, exposure to fresh air is a must especially for those living in large areas.

Breathing techniques are almost always the best way to improve the quality of breathing. Meditation and yoga are great ways of helping in this case. However, the broader issues affecting the nervous system need to be addressed in order to fully guarantee that the person can find the right way to improve their breathing and oxygen absorption.

One other important condition to consider when dealing with vagus nerve-related breathing issues is asthma. While asthma has a clear physiological link to it, the vagus nerve is almost always associated to its worsening or improvement. Hence, is it certainly worth digging deeper into the status of the vagus nerve and addressing any potential issues with it? Experience has shown that improving vagus nerve function has a significant effect in alleviating some of the most debilitating symptoms associated with asthma.

Digestive System Dysfunction

Just like breathing issues, digestive dysfunction is almost a given when the vagus nerve is not functioning to its optimal levels. Since the vagus nerve regulates the digestive system, it is only logical to assume that the vagus nerve needs to be properly tended to in order to ensure that nothing is out of sorts.

Granted, digestive disorders are not exclusively the result of issues with the vagus nerve. There might be a number of reasons why a person would suffer from digestive issues. For instance, digestive issues may be related to physiological causes such as food allergies. It is quite common for people to go for years suffering from poor digestion until they realize that they are allergic to gluten, or some other type of foodstuff.

In other cases, there might be genetic conditions at play such as Crohn's disease. In these cases, dysfunctions of the vagus nerve may serve to aggravate the condition but not actually cause it. Furthermore, treating the vagus nerve would improve the treatment of the condition but not necessarily cure it.

One particular condition that is related to the vagus nerve is gastroparesis. With gastroparesis, it is also common to see Vasovagal Syncope in tandem with this condition.

Gastroparesis is where the stomach cannot void nourishment typically. Actually, it can be defined as a "loss stomach of motion." It can cause acid reflux, queasiness, vomiting, and might be treated with meds or medical procedures. Gastroparesis is a typical condition among individuals who have had diabetes for quite a while however can likewise happen in individuals without diabetes.

It is possible to actually have gastroparesis and not experience any direct symptoms. However, when symptoms do become manifest, the condition may have advanced far enough to where medication is only able to quell them. Here are some of the most common symptoms:

- Stomach distress or swelling (bloating)
- Queasiness
- Alteration of glucose levels
- Feeling full immediately when eating
- Indigestion/Acid Reflux/Gastrointestinal Reflux (GERD)

- Loss of appetite / weight loss / Malnutrition
- Vomiting

Some of these conditions may be indicative of other potential ailments and may not necessarily be traced back to the vagus nerve. But just like in the case of asthma, the vagus nerve can play a significant role in improving the symptoms of the illness as opposed to actually curing them. In that case, it is conceivable that conventional treatments would be enhanced by improving the overall functioning of the vagus nerve.

Dysfunction of the Microbiome

The human gastrointestinal tract has in excess of 100 trillion microscopic organisms and archaea, which together make up the gut microbiota. The measure of microbes in the human gut outnumbers regular human cells by a factor of 10. As such, the human gut microbiota co-advanced with humans to accomplish a harmonious relationship prompting physiological homeostasis. This is a clear example of a symbiotic relationship.

When the gut is out of whack, the body's overall conditioning pays the price. The reason for this is that the microbiota helps digest food and absorb nutrition. When this process does not take place, the body becomes depleted of valuable nutrients. Needless to say, the body needs these little critters in order to fully gain the nutrition it needs.

Dysfunctions and deficiencies in the gut create a condition in which the body cannot fully receive the nutrition it needs. And while we have established that this is partly due to physiological factors which may influence the digestive system, the fact of the matter is that the vagus nerve also plays a critical role insofar as ensuring proper functioning of the body. When the vagus nerve is not at optimal levels, it is quite conceivable that the digestive tract will not be at its best either. The end result is any number of conditions that can arise from improper nutrition.

For example, improper nutrition may result in vitamin deficiency. Deficiency of the B-vitamins may lead to pernicious anemia, nervous system dysfunction and chronic pain. As you can see, it is a feedback loop that fuels itself. That is why it is of the utmost importance to consider gut health as much as possible.

In general, promoting gut health may imply a mix of nutrition such as consuming probiotics such as those found in yogurt. But on the whole, a healthy vagus nerve can go a long way toward setting up a healthy environment for gut health. The most important thing to keep in mind is that the body is an interconnected network meaning that one component cannot fail in isolation. So, if one system falters, the rest of the body will also be affected accordingly.

Cardiac dysfunction

Since the vagus nerve is associated with essential biological functions, the breakdown of this nerve can produce altered heart rhythm. In particular, bradycardia (a slowdown of the heart rate) and tachycardia (an increase in heart rate) may result.

This specific point is completely in concordance with vagus nerve function as this vagus nerve regulates cardiac function. What this entails is that any failure to regulate the heart properly will lead to the conditions mentioned above. Indeed, any potential cardiac failure may result in grave consequences such as a heart attack which can be fatal.

Beyond that, cardiac dysfunction may not necessarily be so serious. But it can be serious enough to leave the sufferer with a significant alteration of their lifestyle. For instance, they may have difficulty engaging in physical activity or may experience chronic fatigue. These symptoms are hardly pleasant and represent a detriment to the quality of life in an individual.

When physiological causes for cardiac problems are discarded, the individual ought to seek proper treatment in order to help correct any dysfunction in their nervous system. This generally implies a reduction of stress and a combination of proper nutrition and relaxation. As you can see, it is the same formula that comes up time and again. Hence, it is important to consider the vital importance that getting away from stressors has on a person's overall health and wellbeing.

Ultimately, maintaining proper cardiac health is a combination of factors that depend largely on proper nervous system management. By now, we have made this point repeatedly. Thus, we sincerely hope that you have already begun to think about ways in which you can begin removing stressors from your life and finding the means to improve your nutrition, exercise and relaxation habits.

Hepatic Dysfunction

Hepatic dysfunction, that is liver dysfunction, may also be traced back to the vagus nerve. While there are clear lifestyle issues that affect liver health, the vagus nerve and its dysfunctions may also play a key role in leading the liver to suffer from abnormal function.

Causes leading to improper liver function are excessive alcohol consumption, increased use of certain prescription medication, a viral infection such as hepatitis and unhealthy eating habits. In such cases, the liver becomes "gunked up". This contamination of the hepatic tissue can lead to further issues starting with digestive problems and moving on to more severe issues such as liver failure.

However, liver dysfunction may also be associated with the vagus nerve. When the vagus nerve is unable to regulate proper digestion, the entire digestive system becomes affected. One of the most common conditions is known as "fatty liver". This condition implies a liver that is so contaminated that it is no longer able to filter any of the substances that are consumed by the body. In that regard, the body progressively becomes intoxicated until it reaches a point where one, or several, organs also begin to show signs of failure. The end result may be the body going into shock. While that may seem extreme, the fact of the matter is that the liver is one of the most important organs in the body. That is why great care needs to be taken to ensure proper hepatic health.

Chronic Stress

We have widely discussed chronic stress throughout this book and its detrimental effect on the nervous system. However, it should be pointed out that chronic stress is just another feedback loop that fuels the feelings of illness and overload that affected the nervous system in the first place. As such, it is a never-ending cycle that leaves the person drained both emotionally and physically. In some cases, chronic stress is one of the leftover byproducts of burnout. Some folks never fully recover from burnout and therefore have to be increasingly careful to avoid falling into the same pattern again.

ADHD and Hyperactivity

ADHD is a neurodevelopmental disorder, which can influence various regions of the brain. It is not an indication of a lack of intelligence or even disability. With proper care and treatment, those with ADHD can effectively overcome the difficulties posed by ADHD. It is highly common in children though it also affects adults.

Folks with ADHD experience:

- Social anxiety
- Difficulty following instructions
- Negligence – experiencing issues concentrating, overlooking guidelines, undertaking one task and then moving onto the next without finishing anything
- Impulsivity – talking over others, having a short attention span, being clumsy
- Sleeping difficulties
- Hyperactivity – consistent eagerness and restlessness
- Inability to carry out complex cognitive tasks due to a lack of concentration and focus

A person coping with ADHD may experience some, or all, of the following:

- Difficulty following rules
- Following through on tasks
- Experience difficulty while playing with other children of the same age group
- experience issues sorting out tasks and exercises
- Being withdrawn as a means of keeping a safe distance between themselves and other children
- A lack of focus and attention to detail especially in schoolwork and other related tasks
- Generally losing things or forgetting where they had been placed.
- Apparent sloppiness and disinterest in neatness
- Appearing not to listen when spoken to directly
- Not begin able to complete tasks such as homework or assigned tasks such as taking care of household chores

There is no conclusive evidence as to the precise reason for ADHD. The main hypothesis is that ADHD is an acquired neurodevelopment disorder. Possible breakdown of the vagus nerve may lead the child to develop inadequately thus leading to the condition. Other contributing factors may include:

- Drugs – consumption of nicotine, alcohol or drugs during pregnancy
- Lead (and other heavy metals) – persistent presence of low degrees of lead may impact conduct and brain science

- Neurophysiology – which incorporates differences in biological systems, electrochemical action in the brain and even gut health

- Absence of early connection – if an infant does not bond with their parent or guardian, or has traumatic experiences identified with connection, this may add to their mindlessness and hyperactivity.
- Hereditary qualities – some examination recommends conceivable quality changes which might be present

A person with post-traumatic stress disorder may have symptoms resembling ADHD, however, it will require different treatment.

Chronic Fatigue Syndrome

Chronic fatigue syndrome (CFS), otherwise called myalgic encephalomyelitis (ME), is an ailment that influences an individual's nervous system (usually called a 'neurological disease'). It can happen at any age and can influence children just like grown-ups.

The term 'myalgic encephalomyelitis' refers to pain in the muscles, and aggravation in the brain and spinal cord. ME/CFS is a disconcerting sickness to which a conclusive origin has not yet been determined. For certain individuals, the condition might be suddenly activated by a viral disease, poisonous agent, sedative, inoculation, gastroenteritis or injury. In other individuals, ME/CFS may grow gradually over months or years.

Around 30 percent of individuals with ME/CFS will have subtle symptoms. Many of these individuals will have the chance to recover rather quickly through a conventional course of treatment. Around 50 percent will have a moderate to a serious case of ME/CFS and not have the option to bounce back quite so quickly. Another 20 percent will encounter serious ME/CFS and need to remain at home or on bedrest until treatment begins to take effect.

There are numerous subtypes within the range of ME/CFS, which implies that a management plan must be created for every individual with the condition. Applying a specific treatment for one subtype can be harming to another subtype. An individual management plan must be produced for every individual with ME/CFS.

Since ME/CFS is an extremely intricate, multi-system, chronic disease, numerous different side effects will happen and should be available for determination. These include:

- Sleeping disorders
- Palpitations, increased pulse or shortness of breath
- Sensitivity to light, smells, contact, sound, food, synthetic compounds, and meds

- Pain or throbbing in the muscles, joints or head
- Inability to adapt to temperature changes

- Gastrointestinal distress, for example, sickness, blockage, bloating or diarrhea
- Issues with cognitive tasks such as concentrating, bad memory, blurry vision, awkwardness, muscle spasms which can also be termed as 'neurocognitive issues'
- Urinary incontinence
- Sore throat, delicate lymph hubs and influenza-like symptoms
- A drop in circulation, dizziness or pale skin
- Sudden fluctuations in weight be it gain or loss

An individual's manifestations will vary over brief timeframes, even from hour to hour.

Chronic fatigue is generally traced back to nervous system overload. In which case, treatment of the vagus nerve may help to alleviate these symptoms or completely reverse them. Therefore, it is definitely a good idea to double-check if there has been any damage to the vagus nerve.

Sleep Issues and Circadian Rhythm Disruption

There are several biological and environmental factors that trigger the brain and cause good or bad sleep. Thus, there are two vital concepts in the human body that trigger the brain and influence a good or bad sleeping experience. Temperature and metabolism influence the level of brain activity since an increase in any of the two leads to an increase in brain activity. Dreams usually occur in the last third of an individual's sleep when brain activity is at its highest. This stage of sleep is known as the Rapid-Eye Movement stage where, depending on their body activity, an individual can experience a bad or good dream.

Foods that rapidly increase the body's metabolism, such as certain condiments and caffeine elevate body temperature and metabolism. In turn, there is an increase in the average brain activity where the individual will take a longer time to move from being fully awake to fast asleep and vice versa. In a similar fashion, any food that adds to the sugar level of the blood, such as sugary foods, increases body temperature and metabolism thereby influencing bad sleep. The increase in the activity of the brain is a consequence of the increase in brain waves.

There are other activities that also trigger brain wave activity causing good or bad quality of sleep. There have been several arguments about the definite influence of sleeping positions in determining the overall quality of sleep. There is evidence to show that poor body positioning and discomfort trigger the brain to produce nightmares and poor sleep. The positioning of the body calls the attention of the brain because of the constant communication it relays with the central nervous system.

For instance, sleeping on the stomach can have significant sway in causing bad sleep in an individual. This is because of the discomfort and strain it places on other body organs and the consequential brain activity through nerve connections. This is why sleeping on your stomach can be uncomfortable since it is plainly uncomfortable and distressing. This is similar to other poor sleeping positions such as sitting upright or having the neck raised too high. Poor body positioning triggers more brain wave activity causing a bad quality of sleep and a lack of rest upon waking.

With that in mind, an overactive nervous system can lead to increased brain wave activity throughout the course of a night's sleep, that is assuming that the individual can get to sleep. This is important to keep in mind as having trouble falling asleep is one of the most common issues that afflict people who are going through issues related to the vagus nerve. In short, addressing any potential issues in the nervous system can go a very long way toward improving sleep quality.

Antisocial Behavior and Lack of Social Interaction

Personality disorders are mental health conditions that influence how somebody thinks, sees, feels or identifies with others. An antisocial personality disorder is an especially testing sort of personality disorder portrayed by hasty, flighty and regularly inappropriate conduct. An individual with an antisocial personality disorder will commonly be manipulative, misleading and neglectful. Moreover, they tend not to take other individuals' feelings into account. Like different sorts of personality disorders, an antisocial personality disorder may range from mild inappropriate social interactions to intermittent improper conduct to overstepping the law and carrying out criminal actions.

Indicators of antisocial behavior include:

- The need to blame others for their shortcomings as opposed to taking personal responsibility
- Lack of concern, lament or regret about other individuals' distress

- Display lack of concern for ordinary social conduct
- Violating the law on a consistent basis
- Experience issues with forming long-term commitment and relationships
- Not being able to control their emotions
- Abuse, control or damage the privileges of others

- Reprimand others for issues in their lives

An individual with antisocial character disorder will have a past filled with lead disorder during youth, for example, skipping school (not going to class), wrongdoing (for instance, carrying out violations or substance abuse), and other troublesome and forceful practices.

PART III: THE MIND BODY CONNECTION

Chapter 7: The Physical and Emotional Connection Between the Mind and the Body

In ancient Greece, three specialists would see a patient in tandem. They were the "knife" specialist, the "herb" specialist, and the "language" specialist. The individuals who "designed" medication comprehended there was an association between the mind and body and functioned in a similar manner. Our cutting-edge Western doctors (specialists, physicians, and pharmacists) will only occasionally talk with one another regarding the specific course of treatment for a patient.

There is expanding proof the ancient Greeks were correct: our considerations, feelings, and states of mind can influence how our organism works. Also, what we do with our physical bodies can influence our psychological state. Indeed, until around 300 years ago, most conventional medical treatments regarded the mind and body only in a general sense. It was not until the seventeenth century that Western societies started to consider the possibility of the mind playing a role in physical maladies. Analysts started going back to the mind-body association in the late twentieth century, and from that point forward, there has been a noteworthy increase in the amount of information that evidences how our bodies and minds share a common linguistic framework as they are always speaking to each other.

Prolonged exposure to stress can emerge from events such as worry about a friend or family member's wellbeing and health, living in perilous conditions, financial considerations, unrealistic demands in the workplace, and so on. The experience of prolonged periods of stress causes an increase in heart rate, inappropriate breathing, muscle pain and discomfort, and circulatory issues, among many of the physical ailments we have discussed. Most side effects of incessant stress are physical such as migraines, stomachaches, muscle pain, sleep problems, chest pain, weakness, changes in sex drive among others. We have also explored the mental and emotional issues that arise such as anxiety, depression, and even antisocial behavior. Stress likewise causes increased production of the cortisol hormone which analysts have connected to medical issues such as weight gain, insulin resistance, and even cognitive decline.

Perhaps the most evident impact of incessant stress, which we frequently consider as an illness itself, is anxiety. Since our bodies are intended to deal with smaller doses of mental and emotional stress, it is vital for us to remain focused on our surroundings in order to deal with any situations that may arise at any given point. In any case, if we are not prepared to deal with prolonged stress, we may face a considerable uphill battle when looking to maintain proper mind-body balance.

It is crucial that we perceive the association between our bodies and psyches if we intend to feel our best. If you happen to feel anything less than your absolute vest, you might want to visit your primary care physician to check nutrient levels and screen for thyroid or gastrointestinal issues. Specialists could consider persistent stress as a risk to wellbeing and urge patients to talk with a licensed therapist when needed.

With that in mind, physicians need to work in tandem with therapists in order to uncover the causes of inexplicable illnesses that may be afflicting a patient. This is often the case when a battery of tests has been run and there are no discernible causes that can explain the ailments of the patient. In short, achieving full health and wellbeing is not just a matter of seeing your doctor and taking meds, it is also a matter of digging a bit deeper into your overall psychological and emotional state.

One of the most extraordinary concepts on how constant stress can influence the body is called "broken heart disorder."

The experience of stress, because of a broken relationship, or even divorce, can cause significant amounts of stress for prolonged periods of time to a point where the individual may end up completely exhausted, both physically and emotionally. Indeed, prolonged exposure to such circumstances may prompt cardiovascular breakdown and even cognitive decline. The New England Journal of Medicine published a study on hormones such as adrenaline, noradrenaline, and cortisol discharged in the body, in abnormally high amounts, as a result of prolonged stress or anguish, in which the guilty party was identified as broken heart disorder. Specialists discovered treating this sort of cardiovascular breakdown with customary pharmacology would not be viable, though psychotherapy focusing on managing feelings and expectations helped alleviate the worst parts of the symptoms.

Based on the previous discussion, we can see how stress is an incredibly powerful force that can impact a person in a myriad of ways. In fact, most of the physical ailments that a person can manifest may be traced, one way or another, to emotional and psychological issues. These issues may have their roots in childhood, or they may be unresolved issues that have lingered and subsequently festered over time. The fact of the matter is that these physical manifestations are the living embodiment of the mind-body connection. Hence, attempting to ignore this relationship is a futile task. We must acknowledge the fact that the connection that exists between both aspects of the human condition make it crucial to develop a working knowledge of this connection.

Given the fact that the nervous system is connected to the brain, which is believed to the be organ closest related to thought and emotion, we can clearly see the connection between our feelings and our emotions and how the body can begin to express the manifestation of these feelings. This is a clear indication that there is a direct causal link between what the mind feels and what the body manifests at various levels. As such, there is no doubt that we cannot ignore the role the mind plays in overall health and wellness any longer.

However, most physicians will first attempt to discover the underlying physical causes of illness. After all, physicians are trained to do so. But often, physicians ignore the role that the mind plays in maintaining health or breaking it down. And just like the mind can cause illness, the mind can also heal. This is a very important assumption to keep in mind as the mind-body connection is indisputable. The body of research in this area is consistently growing. As a result, we cannot ignore that there is a divide between the mind and the body. In fact, the time has come for us to embrace the fact that our thoughts are just as likely to heal us as they are to hurt us.

With that in mind, it's worth digging deeper into the connections among other body systems and the mind. For instance, the connection between the mind and the gut, while often overlooked, are clear and coherent. When the mind is free of stress, the gut reacts accordingly, and vice versa. Yet, it is far more often that the mind affects the gut than the other way around. When the gut is ill, that affects the rest of the body. Consequently, the body enters a negative feedback loop in which it is unable to rid itself of the persistent ill effects of being sick. Rather, it enters a cycle in which it only fuels the patterns that are causing it to be sick in the first place. This is why we need to address this issue in closer detail.

Chapter 8: How the Mind Talks to the Gut

Ever "gone with your gut" when settling on a choice?

You are most likely accepting a sign from your gastrointestinal tract, which discusses, literally, with your brain. Constant digestive distress has been down to reduce cognitive ability and generate positive feelings. When we become debilitated with conditions like intestinal infection, our brains become reworked through a procedure called neuroplasticity, which changes the associations between the nerve signals among the various interconnect systems.

Stress can impact the sort of microscopic organisms possessing the gut, making our gut configuration less favorable and progressively allowing hurtful microbes to take a foothold. It can likewise build irritation in the gut and break down immunity to contamination and even allergies to certain foodstuffs.

The brain and gut address each other through a system of neural, hormonal and immunological messages on a consistent basis. In any case, this solid correspondence can be exasperating when we are under stress or experience constant digestive distress in the digestive system.

Due to the amount of nerve endings and transmitters that exist in the gut, it is called the "second brain". There is good reason to make this claim as the amount of information that is processed in the gut enables the body to repair itself, absorb nutrients and provide the brain with the necessary elements it requires for the overall functioning of the body's various biological systems.

As such, this ongoing dialogue between the brain and the gut means that there is a direct link between the CNS and the digestive system. Moreover, if we consider the fact that the brain is the main processing center where the mind manifests itself, then there is no doubt that the link between the mind and the gut is very much real.

This brings us back to the point about the mind being able to both make the body ill and heal it. This proposition picks up significant steam when considering the existence of so-called psychosomatic illnesses. These illnesses have their roots in psychological and emotional causes as opposed to purely physiological ones. When these causes are explored, usually after deep periods of introspection, a root cause may be identified. When the root cause is identified, the psychological burden can begin to be lifted off the nervous system and eventually dissipate the stress and anxiety that may be accompanying the individual everywhere they go.

Upon closer examination, this causal link between mind, feelings, and gut truly gives credence to the notion that there is such a thing as "gut feelings". While some may argue that gut feelings are a figurative way of explaining the role of intuition in the life of humans, it is certainly worth examining at a closer level. Gut feelings are often associated as unconscious choices that individuals make, not based on facts or evidence, but rather on assumptions and guesswork. The likelihood of being right on these hunches is, at best, 50/50. This idea is more the product of the law of probability more than any reasonable assertation. In truth, the fact that we, as humans, have the extraordinary ability to intuit things without rationally thinking them through is more the product of perception and clarity than any supernatural ability. Nevertheless, the gut does play a pivotal role in this endeavor as it serves as a secondary processing unit. And while the gut does not produce articulated thought in the same manner the brain does, it does provide enough data for the brain to arrive at a reasonable conclusion even if it doesn't seem perfectly understandable at the time.

So, the next time you experience a "gut feeling" ask yourself what's really on your mind. It could be that the feelings you are perceiving are more of a manifestation of underlying thoughts and even repressed feelings that have yet to surface at a reasonable moment. Therefore, your gut will tell you far more than you could have ever thought possible based solely on your intellectual processes.

Chapter 9: About Gut Feelings

What is Gut Instinct?

A large portion of us has encountered the feeling of knowing things before we know them, regardless of whether we cannot clarify how. You delay at a green light and miss getting hit by a speeding truck. You settle spontaneously to break your no-arranged meetings strategy and end up gathering your life accomplice. You suspect that you ought to put resources into a little online startup and it progresses toward becoming Google.

As indicated by numerous analysts, instinct is undeniably quite material. The natural right brain is quite often "perusing" your environment, in any event, when your cognizant left brain is generally locked in, the body can enlist this data while the cognizant personality remains willfully ignorant of what's happening.

So, as we have discussed earlier, does it mean that you can truly intuit things around you without consciously having to process them? Turns out you can, particularly if you figure out how to identify which signs to concentrate on — regardless of whether they are sweat-soaked palms, a strong feeling in the pit of your stomach, or an unexpected and incomprehensible conviction that something is going on. These may all be subconscious manifestations coming from your "second brain", but that somehow the "first brain" is unable to process consciously.

Another hypothesis purports you can actually feel chemical changes in your brain as they occur. This may explain why some folks can literally describe their thought process as it is happening. Others may be able to pick up on these processes but may be unable to articulate them in an intelligible manner. While this doesn't mean that these folks are somehow less intelligent, it does mean that others are more in tune with their feelings and how to express them in a more articulated manner.

This implies if something in the earth is even marginally perceptible — the speed of a moving toward the truck, the somewhat bizarre conduct of somebody at a gathering — your mind can somehow pick up the chemical changes in your brain which leads to that "abnormal" feeling. Regardless of whether you focus or not can have a significant effect. You may meet your future life partner — or meet your new boss. Those signs convey a great deal of significant data, so it is wise to hone these skills. In a way, this is more about perception of reality than anything else you could potentially do.

The advantages of tuning in to your senses go a long way past following through on life-or-passing choices. Living all the more naturally requests that you are at the time and that makes for an increasingly energetic life.

In any case, gut impulses are a long way from dependable. The brain's expertise based on fact and evidence can trigger doubts of new (however not hazardous) things or cause you to be particularly receptive to individuals who essentially help you to remember another person.

So, how would you pick which gut feelings to trust? It is a matter of "going along to get along" and finding some kind of harmony between gut intuition and normal reasoning. When you have seen a logical connection, you can draw on the sensible side of your personality to gauge your decisions and choose how best to follow up on them.

After all, there is no reason why you shouldn't trust your gut instincts unless you can be sure that they are wrong. Of course, there are plenty of stories out there of people who went against their better judgment and trusted their instincts. However, their stories are not nearly as common as those in which the protagonists happen to miss the mark by following their hunches.

Again, this point is not meant to discredit the merits of hunches and instincts. If anything, we should all be in tune with our feelings in such a way that we are able to recognize when something deeper inside of us is trying to tell us that something isn't quite right. Perhaps you get a sudden urge to do something that you normally wouldn't. All of those manifestations of intuition largely depend on what we are able to perceive long before it actually happens.

One contending theory is that when both the brain and the gut are in good health, they are both able to combine their processing power. This means that the sensory information that enters the body is processed by the brain with the aid of the gut. As a result, you are able to perceive situations before they happen thus giving credibility to the notion that you can intuit things without necessarily being aware of them.

Based on the previous premise, if your gut and brain both combine to process information which was not previously available, then it is safe to say that you "know" things before the brain is actually able to arrive to a logical conclusion. The truth is that you are generally able to rationalize the events that occurred after the fact, meaning that in hindsight, you are able to make sense of why your guess was right. In any event, you have the opportunity to dissect what happened and therefore come to a conclusion as to why you were right, or perhaps why you wrong.

At the end of the day, when you improve your gut health, you are giving your cognitive power a significant boost insofar as being able to combine the processing power that is within your body. When all systems are humming at the optimal capacity, you are then able to really make sense of the world around you even if you aren't always consciously aware of why things are the way they are.

Hence, don't be afraid to go on a hunch especially if it doesn't seem to contradict your better judgment right at once. Of course, it might be that you can find logical inconsistencies with the hunch once you drill down and look at the deficiencies in your thought patterns. But that doesn't mean that you should discard your feelings off hand. It could be that your body is trying to tell you something that you know at a deeper level but may be reluctant to accept at a more conscious level.

Chapter 10: How the Gut Talks to the Brain

The article "Digestive Distress: A Civilization Disorder" by Watson and Collins, provides intriguing insights into the prevalence of digestive disorders. The authors of the article focus on providing information about the differences that are present in women and men when contracting the disease. According to research from the authors, women display higher rates of infection than in men in several countries. The biological differences in the make-up of the body of a man and woman result in different effects on the digestive system. The authors highlight the fact that the disease is a significant disruption to civilization as it is responsible for several deaths. The community is slowly being disintegrated as a result of the prevalence of harmful diseases such as digestive disorders that are usually preventable. The article analyzes different causes of the disease and offers the insight of the authors as appropriate recommendations to follow.

The article also provides information about the different types of cancers responsible for a high number of deaths. The authors ensure that they provide appropriate information by referencing different scientific studies from institutions around the world. The findings of the authors are accurate and precise in describing the harmful consequence of digestive disorders in society. There is information about the awareness program in the United States that educates the population on the dangers of digestive diseases. There is a strong emphasis by the authors on insisting that women change their eating habits for the sake of preventing digestive disorders among other digestive disorders. The biological differences between both sets of the population mean that women need to exercise greater caution than their male counterparts in preventing the prevalence of the disease. The authors conclude by suggesting that digestive disorders have the potential of increasing its scope and harm in society if no appropriate control measures are implemented.

While there may be clear differences in the propensity to certain types of cancer according to gender, it is important to note that gut health and the broader digestive system can break down in equal proportion to men and women. As such, it is worth considering the following guidelines when looking to protect how the gut and brain communicate especially with the heightened risk of cancer among other potential illnesses.

Diet

The diet solutions of most people in society are perhaps the most significant cause of digestive issues. Poor nutrition, inadequate diets and the increase in pollutants in the body is accredited to diet as a cause of all sorts of digestive maladies in human beings. The body requires adequate nutrients and the right balance of food in order for all the organs to function properly. Any inadequacies result in the failure of some body organs and unfavorable biological reactions that may result in serious illness such as digestive disorders. The food in the modern world certainly does not help in allowing the population to retains high levels of health. A majority of the manufactured food products have a high amount of chemicals and other dangerous, unnatural substances that damage the body. Maintaining a healthy and strict diet is a difficult responsibility for most people living in the modern world with several alternative food products available to try.

Doctors and physicians around the world have let it be known that a majority of patients suffer as a result of their own actions. The high consumption of dangerous foods continuously results in bodily damage in the intestines. Some of these food products also prevent the body from carrying out essential functions, such as metabolism and the removal of waste. The accumulation of these harmful substances in the body causes massive cell and gene mutations. The colon is most vulnerable as it pays the primary responsibility of absorbing water for the body. The poor dieting regimes of most people in spite of them thinking that they are eating healthily result in digestive disorders. The dieting regimes of each individual require thorough scrutiny if digestive disorders are going to permanently disappear from the community. The digestive disorders awareness month in the United States aims at encouraging healthy diets to the population as a way of averting this disease in the community.

Fiber

Fiber plays an extremely important role in the digestion of food and nutrients in the human body. In terms of consumption, there are two different types of fiber than are accessible through nutrition. First, soluble fiber can be digested in the body through the normal process of digestion. Secondly, insoluble fiber is that which cannot be digested but instead passes through the gut. It is vital to note that fiber primarily comes from plants alone; it is not possible to acquire this essential nutrient from meat and other such sources. The absence of soluble fiber in the diet of an individual contributes greatly to the prevalence of digestive disorders in their lives. This is because this nutrient is responsible for reducing the levels of cholesterol in the blood, limiting the potential of an increase in body fat.

Individuals who consume high amounts of soluble fiber remain relatively healthier than those who consume high amounts of red meat and alcohol. Biologically, soluble fiber contributes directly to the digestion process as it allows for the easier absorption of nutrients in the body. The sources of soluble fiber include oats, barley, rye, fruits, root vegetables such as carrots and potatoes and golden linseeds. Insoluble fiber, however, cannot be digested and moves down the gut to help other foods move more easily in the digestive system. They are responsible for keeping the digestive system clean and healthy and contribute tremendously towards weight loss. Diets that have little or inadequate soluble and insoluble fiber are responsible for causing a high prevalence of digestive disorders in the human body. The credible sources of insoluble fiber that can help in reducing the chances of this cancer include bran, wholemeal bread, cereals, seeds, and nuts.

The Mouse Model

The research on the gnotobiotic mouse model shows that digestive disorders are preventable by relying on dietary fiber. Conflicting epidemiological findings suggest that dietary fiber does not protect against digestive disorders. Experiments that involved using mice, however, demonstrate that fiber is pivotal in the prevention of digestive disorders. In the experiment, scientists would monitor the digestion of fiber in the mice and analyze the effect of the hormones and proteins. In their findings, the gut microbiota is responsible for fermenting the fiber into short-chain fatty acids such as butyrate. The fatty acids would offer protection to the internal colon lining of the mice and limits the potential of the growth and expansion of abnormal cells. The butyrate accomplishes this by preventing the accumulation of β-catenin protein to hazardous levels. The breakdown of the fiber in the mice is an excellent example of the role that fiber plays in reducing the instances of digestive disorders.

Meat

Red meat is much more harmful than white meat in controlling digestive disorders. Scientific evidence shows that high consumption of red meats increases the chances of digestive disorders in individuals. Moderate consumption of this meat is instrumental in individuals who have never experienced the disease. The common sources of this diet include lamb, beef and liver, and it causes serious health problems in individuals when consumed in high amounts. The danger that these food options pose is also evident in processed meats such as bologna, hot dogs and lunch meat. White meats are better alternatives as diets and a source of nutrition because they do not have a high percentage of cholesterol than their counterparts. The continuous consumption of this option instead of red meat prevents the sudden gain of weight that is a common characteristic of red meat diets.

High cholesterol levels in the body encourage the release of insulin. This hormone directly contributes to the growth of cancerous cells in the colon by making conditions favorable for the mutant cells. The methods of cooking meat also reveal the flaws of this diet option in encouraging the prevalence of digestive disorders. Scientific evidence shows that cooking meat at very high heat temperatures can be hazardous for the digestive system. relationship is because the heat can create chemicals in the process of cooking that increase the chances of contracting digestive disorders. Broiling, frying or grilling attracts the mixture of the meat with various chemicals at high temperatures. The situation is worsened in the case of processed meats that already have preservative chemicals in them. Consuming meat that is prepared using these methods for long periods of time leaves the victim vulnerable to consuming pollutants and suffering from digestive disorders.

The lifestyle and dietary options of the community are going to be influential in determining the prevalence of digestive disorders. As long as there is a tendency to enjoy a life of opulence without careful regard for the health consequences will result in an increase in digestive disorders cases. Doctors and physicians from around the world are insisting on the importance of revolutionizing the feeding habits of all human communities. The reliance on foods that have high percentages of sugars and fats attracts the possibility of lifestyle diseases in the population and compromises the health of everybody.

Children in schools need to be given appropriate advice and adequate information on their lifestyle choices. It is possible to completely eliminate the threat caused by digestive disorders by ensuring everybody is aware of the importance of living a healthy lifestyle. Starting this education in earnest from an early age will allow future generations to live much more healthy lives and experience higher life expectancy ratios. There is a possibility of eliminating digestive disorders in society, along with the other dangerous types of cancer responsible for millions of deaths across the globe. Education, awareness and proper dieting are the ways of guaranteeing a much healthier community.

How Communication Takes Places

When everything is humming along just fine, the neuroreceptors in the gut are free to communicate adequately with the rest of the body. In particular, the ongoing dialogue between the gut and the brain takes place through the vagus nerve. It is the vagus nerve that ends up facilitating this communicating since it mainly serves as a large highway for information to flow to and from. As a result, the brain is keenly aware of what's going in the gut and the gut is keenly aware of what the brain is attempting to communicate.

When this dialogue is fostered by proper nutrition and the removal of damaging foods, the gut is even able to repair itself. This also leads to the overall health of the nervous system and vice versa. In fact, we've talked so much about how negative feedback loops are created in the body. Now, in this particular case, we can focus on positive feedback since a healthy nervous system promotes a healthy gut while a healthy gut promotes a healthy nervous system. This interaction is a manner of give and take. In the end, the body is perfectly balanced with the rest of the biological systems.

At the end of the day, the body is able to tell the difference between foreign substances that might be potentially harmful and give the immune system a leg up. This is why you find that certain people are much healthier than others. After all, when you stop overloading your body, you are able to let it act freely. When it has the freedom to attack what it should be attacking, then you can truly focus on being healthy. Moreover, when you eliminate harmful foods from your diet, the body is no long tasked with helping the digestive system deal with harmful substances in food; the immune system and digestive tract are all focused on being ready to do their job.

So, this is why cleaning up your diet as much as possible is absolutely vital to ensuring that you have everything you need to make your life that much better. You can certainly improve your quality of life by improving your eating habits and fostering a positive communication link between your gut and brain.

Chapter 11: How to Improve Brain-Gut Health

A solid gut, which houses a fair microbiome, is increasingly impervious to the negative effects of inescapable stress. Omega-3 unsaturated fats, fat-dissolvable nutrients An and D, and adjusted probiotics would all be able to help recuperate the intestinal coating, lessen irritation, and give various exhibits of useful microorganisms. This makes your stomach related tract stronger to the destructive effects of stress.

Investigate What Your Digestive Symptoms Can Teach You

Your digestive system can be seen as an indicator of how you are adapting to life. Stomach related indications frequently give understanding into the base of what is causing your stress, enabling you to push toward recuperating. On the contrary, if you cannot detect any abnormalities, then you can be sure that you aren't suffering from any major conditions.

For instance, if you are inclined to obstruction you may investigate where in life you cannot give up. If you have constant acid reflux, you may take a gander at where you may feel you have been "scorched" or where you are clutching resentment or disdain. Investigating your stomach related indications from this figurative point of view can enable you to see your feelings, process them, and discharge them so you can more readily adapt to stress. Indeed, this is an approximation to the psychosomatic effects that mental anguish has on the body's physical manifestations.

Whenever you see a gut feeling or your digestive system is acting up, respect this shrewd system by focusing on what may go on in your life. When you figure out how to comprehend your feelings and reactions to stress and receive sound approaches to oversee stress, you can all the more adequately digest both nourishment and life.

Keep away from Negativity to Heal Your Gut

Negative considerations are an enormous supporter of stress in the current life. Figuring out how to perceive your considerations through care or other contemplation methods enables you to change your attitude. This diminishes ceaseless stress yet can likewise enable you to settle on more advantageous nourishment decisions that improve absorption. Uneasiness, despondency, and other uncertain feelings are regularly at the foundation of indulging and poor nourishment decisions that can further stress processing.

Energy and empathy improve the capacity of the vagus nerve, which is vital in the correspondence between the brain and stomach related system. Practices, for example, adoring benevolence contemplation can expand your confidence, which thusly balances the nervous system and decidedly influence processing. It definitely goes without saying that whenever you can positively charge yourself, you will be having a positive effect on your entire body. Your body feeds off your positive energy in the exact same manner your entire biological framework is affected by negative energy. As a result, you must make a point of cutting out as much negative energy as you can. Otherwise, you may find yourself contaminating your body with needless rubbish that may only lead you to further detriment. A wise choice is to focus on your loved ones and the experiences which leave you feeling better about life and yourself. It may be high time to do some house cleaning for the sake of better gut health.

PART IV: STIMULATING THE VAGUS NERVE

Chapter 11: The Benefits of Vagus Nerve Stimulation

Throughout this book, we have talked about the importance of caring for the vagus nerve. We have clearly established the reasons why the vagus nerve is so important and the negative consequences of ignoring its wellbeing. At this point, the time has come to discuss the ways in which the vagus nerve can better serve the body's overall wellbeing. In this chapter, we are going to focus on the benefits that you can derive from stimulating the vagus nerve in a positive manner.

Firstly, it should be noted that the key concept in vagus nerve stimulation is the reduction of stress on the nervous system. This begins with calming and soothing the CNS while allowing the PNS to do its job. When this occurs, a great deal of the stress and pressure on the vagus nerve is reduced. As a result, the vagus nerve can recover and eventually restore the proper balance in the entire body's systems.

A Natural Way to Stimulate the Vagus Nerve

The most common technique used to calm the nervous system is meditation. Now, meditation doesn't have to be a complex endeavor. In fact, most folks who are unfamiliar with meditation believe it to be some sort of mystical art that must be practiced atop a mountain.

The truth is that meditation can be practiced anywhere at any time. The key point to meditation is to free the mind from thought. This does not mean that the mind must be completely blank; that is virtually impossible What this means is that the mind must be free of those thoughts which cause it to fixate on negative aspects. For instance, if you are overly concerned about paying the rent at the end of the month, this fixation may lead you to lose sleep, eat poorly and become anxious at various points throughout the day. When you apply meditation to the mix, you can allow your mind the break the shackles of worry and even come up with solutions to the problems afflicting you.

The easiest way in which you can practice meditation is to take 5 or 10 minutes of your time and just close your eyes. When you attempt to relax, try deep breathing. This will allow enough air to enter your lungs. As your blood becomes rich in oxygen, the nervous system suddenly becomes energized by the rush of fresh air. If you happen to feel that you are becoming anxious, you can retreat to a "happy place". While that may should cheesy, it actually works. This tenet behind a happy place is that you are stimulating positive feelings. As a result, positive feelings become positive energy. When positive energy begins to permeate your body, you will be able to literally feel this vibe enveloping your body.

As you become more and more proficient with meditation, you will begin to see the following benefits:

1.	Reduced anxiety

When you practice meditation, you often find that anxiety is reduced simply because you are able to shift your focus away from what is ailing you. Even if it is making a relentless assault on your conscious thought, you have the power to divert these negative thoughts into more positive means. For example, your meditation may consist of positive visualization in which you see yourself actually being successful at something. This visualization technique is so effective due to its simplicity. You don't need to do anything special; just breathe and imagine yourself achieving whatever you want to achieve.

2.   Increased blow flow and circulation

Another benefit is the improvement of circulation in your body. When you are able to focus on diverting your mind from negative thought, the blood in your veins begins to flow more freely especially since the blood vessels begin to feel less constricted. This effect is often described as a warm feeling all over. This sensation of blood going through your veins is equal to having a strenuous workout. When you push yourself physically, your heart begins to pump blood quite forcefully. The end result is your circulation improving. The same effect can be achieved when the nervous system relaxes and focuses on regulating essential biological functions.

3.   Decreased heart rate

If you find that your heart is racing all the time especially when you think about all of the things on your plate, your heart rate begins to pick up. On the flip side, if you are able to focus your attention on other, more positive thoughts, your mind then begins to shift the focus from stress and on positive energy. This gives your vagus nerve a much-deserved break to the point where it no longer pushes the heart to beat faster. Rather, the vagus nerve can focus on restoring the heart's proper rate. When this happens, you can literally feel your body begin to slow down. This, on top of proper circulation, will lead your cardiovascular system to achieve its optimal level of functioning.

4.   Improved immune response

When the body is no longer overloaded with worry and concern, the immune system is able to take a step back a catch a breather. At this point, some folks claim that they get sick with a common illness like a cold or the flu. The fact of the matter is that when the immune system is not forced into overdrive, what it does it that it actually fights off bugs that might be in your system. However, your overexcited state may not allow you to actually feel sick. This is nothing more than a consequence of an excited state that keeps the individual going on pure adrenaline. When your immune system is able to take five, you will find that you no longer get sick as often, and when you do, your illness is not nearly a tough to deal with as it had otherwise been.

5.   Better cognitive ability

Perhaps the biggest benefit of improving the vagus nerve is the overall boost to your cognitive abilities. When you manage to get worry and anxiety out of your system, you are able to free up valuable real estate in your brain so that you can dedicate it to the tasks that you actually need to get done. This is manifest in better grades in school, improved performance at work, or simply being able to focus more on the things which you normally do.

In addition to meditation, mindfulness is one of the best ways in which you can unlock the above-mentioned benefits. Mindfulness is a state in which you are living in the here and now. When you enter a mindful state, you are giving your mind the leeway it needs to think about the task at hand rather than worrying about whatever is on your mind. Sure, this may not solve the problem at hand, but it will at least you give some peace of mind while in the mindful state.

Chapter 12: Vagus Nerve Stimulation Techniques and Exercises

Microbiotic and probiotic manipulation is a new-found science that will be instrumental in the treatment of various diseases, particularly those that affect the Central Nervous System. The 'gut-brain axis' refers to the association between the gastrointestinal system and the central nervous system (CNS), which has been increasingly looked upon as a sort of symbiotic relationship in the body and is now seen as a possible avenue for treatment of CNS disorders. The gut-brain axis is an insightful approach towards solving health and medical problems associated with a breakdown in the Central Nervous System in the human body.

This approach has been discussed as a revolutionary approach towards treating different conditions that affect the Central Nervous System in the human body. Microbiotic and probiotic manipulation in the human body is important in treating and preventing multiple diseases that have long been associated with the nervous system. There is a clear link between gastrointestinal health and CNS disorders such as ASD that brings forth relevance to the manipulation process as a method of treatment. This method is gaining popularity among health care practitioners as they seek the most effective ways of addressing some of the problems experienced by their patients via the Central Nervous System.

The purpose of this form of treatment is to restore the neurological pathways in the central nervous system destroyed by disease. There is a rapidly increasing amount of evidence implicating host-microbe interactions at virtually all levels of complexity, ranging from direct cell-to-cell communication to extensive systemic signaling, and involving various organs and organ systems, including the central nervous system (CNS). This treatment approach is critical to getting the most appropriate method of implementing a relevant remedy for the central nervous system.

Self-healing through Yoga

Yoga exercises are ancient Indian practices that serve the critical purpose of 'uniting the body, mind, and spirit.' The essence of yoga exercises is to strike a perfect balance within the nervous system that puts the entire body at ease. Practicing yoga exercises on a constant basis is a good way of staying in shape and reducing stress, particularly in work environments where people spend significant portions of their time.

The yoga exercises prescribed are my personal favorite because I engage in them at least once a day. The exercises have become a tradition because they are effective ways of changing mood and feelings of exhaustion. When working behind a desk for several hours, energy levels wane and stress easily kicks in. Performing various stretches as prescribed in yoga for just a few minutes can work wonders by completely clearing the head.

STEP-BY-STEP process

1.   Forward Bend

The first technique, the "Forward Bend", involves stretching the back and allowing the tension on the neck to disappear. The technique involves the individual first standing upright, then bending forward and allowing your knees to bend. The feet- hip-distance must remain reasonable and the individual should remain in this pose for six full breaths. Thereafter, fold the legs and hold down your head, shaking it first for six full breaths, and then nodding for six full breaths. The entire process should take no more than a few minutes, but it helps ensure that blood circulation is distributing an adequate amount of oxygen to the rest of the body.

2.   Eagle Arms

Shoulder knots can be quite frustrating, particularly for those who spend most of their time hunched over a desk. The 'Eagle Arms' technique involves standing upright with the arms outward and parallel to the ground. Swing the arms, and then bend the elbows to the extent that the back of the hands can touch each other. Thereafter, hook the right arm over the left so that they are facing each other directly, remain in this position looking straight ahead and maintain the position of the elbows. Slowly pull the elbows apart as the shoulders remain relaxed, remaining in this position for five breaths then unwrap the arms and swing them together.

3.   Band Stretch

The "Band Stretch" is another yoga exercise that involves completely laying down on the ground and stretching the legs. Begin by bending the left leg, with the left foot flat on the ground and then put your right foot on top of the left knee. Put your arms around the left thigh while pulling it towards you, stretching the hips on the right side. Remain in this position for a few breaths, and then switch up the process by starting over by bending the right leg to stretch the hips on the left side.

4.	Square Breathing

"Square Breathing" is a straightforward yoga exercise that involves taking deep breaths as a remedy for clearing the mind and de-stressing. The biological process of breathing accounts for a significant part of brain activity because constant oxygen is needed for this vital organ. The technique must begin with the individual sitting upright and inhaling through the nose deeply and holding that breath. Thereafter, exhale through the nose, timing no more than five seconds on each occasion and allowing the air to move indiscriminately. Repeat the cycle a few more times as it supplies more oxygen to the brain and hastens the process of carbon dioxide exhalation, de-stressing the individual.

5.	Heart Opener

The "Heart Opener" is another yoga exercise technique that is particularly effective for the chest region. While standing, reach the arms towards the back with the feet hip-distance apart, then hook the hands together at the base of the back. Slowly lift the hooked hands behind you, allowing them to stretch the shoulder blades as the body tilts and bends over. Remain in this position for about a minute as it reduces stress by stretching the back and allowing for effective blood circulation in the body.

6.   Shoulder Stretch

The "Shoulder Stretch" is the last yoga technique that is applicable for a wide range of purposes. Interlock the fingers and raise the hands above the head facing upwards, ensuring the hands remain in line with the ears. While looking ahead, relax the shoulder blades and remain in this position for five full breaths, then allowing the arms to fall on the sides. Take deep breaths through the nose while conducting the stretch as it increases the rate at which oxygen is being absorbed by the blood and the vice-versa expulsion of carbon dioxide. This process reduces stress because it relaxes the shoulders and allows for the relaxation of the back.

The prescribed yoga stretches can be performed almost anywhere, even at work. The best time to perform these exercises is at the peak of activity when a break is needed. Taking some time off to conduct different body stretches helps to clear up the mind by boosting the circulation of oxygen in the body. This traditional Indian technique has been adopted by peoples from all over the world for its effectiveness in reducing stress. Yoga techniques are several in their types and sometimes depend on the physical fitness of the individual, but overall, they are particularly helpful. The breathing processes involved in yoga are the most essential aspect of the exercises because all the body parts work in tandem to reduce stress and instances of fatigue than an individual might experience.

A majority of the stretches are highly reliant on loosening the body and moving the limbs as freely as possible. Clothing must be taken into consideration when performing yoga exercises because tight jeans and skirts might not be appropriate for some of the stretches. Some of the stretches that involve completely laying on the ground must also be taken into consideration because they might be disruptive to the people in a work environment. The essence of yoga exercises is to reduce stress in the individual and restoring excellent oxygen circulation is a pivotal element of yoga exercises. The stretches become effective and successful to those who engage in it and find themselves stress-free if they develop a timetable and make it a routine in their daily lives.

Chapter 13: The Polyvagal Theory

Polyvagal theory clarifies three different pieces of our nervous system and their reactions to stressful circumstances. When we comprehend those three sections, we can perceive any reason why and how we respond to high measures of stress.

Polyvagal theory is an innovative approach that serves to stimulate the vagus nerve thereby unlocking its potential while repairing any damage that may have come to it. It is a captivating clarification of how our body handles stress, and how we can utilize different treatments it to revise the impact of injury.

Why is polyvagal theory significant?

For specialists, and psychology science lovers, too, understanding polyvagal theory can help with:

- Understanding significant mood swings
- Seeing how to peruse someone using body language
- Getting through physical injury and conditions such as PTSD
- Seeing how extraordinary stress prompts separation or even shutdown

We like to think about our feelings as ethereal, complex, and difficult to classify and identify.

In all actuality, feelings are reactions to an upgrade (inward or outer). Frequently they occur out of our mindfulness, particularly if we are distant, or incongruent, with our inward passionate life.

The nervous system is continually running out of sight, controlling our body's capacities so we can consider different things — like what sort of frozen yogurt we'd like to order, or how to get an "A" in school. The whole nervous system works with the brain and can assume control over our enthusiastic experience, regardless of whether we do not need it to.

Our basic want to remain alive is more essential to our body than even our capacity to consider remaining alive. That is the place the polyvagal theory comes in to play. In this next chapter, we are going to be taking a look at how you can put Polyvagal theory to the test.

Chapter 14: The Healing Power of Polyvagal Theory

The polyvagal theory depicts three neural circuits that underlie different methods for consulting with our condition. When we have a sense of security, we depend upon a neural circuit that advances social commitment practices. He calls this the social nervous system. This piece of the parasympathetic nervous system draws in neural structures that restrain our guarded systems. This depends upon the myelinated ventral vagus nerve which enables us to connect socially by looking, relaxing our voice tone, and communicating care with our face. Significantly, the social nervous system can encourage immobilization inside setting security to advance more noteworthy closeness or closeness.

At first, when we experience a risk, we may depend upon our social nervous system to determine the circumstance. We may connect for association or nearness with another to restore security. In any case, if this is fruitless or if the risk is progressively extraordinary, we will start to draw in the sympathetic nervous system initiation of battle or flight.

If we cannot resolve the compromising circumstance by battling or escaping then we will start to draw in an unmyelinated, developmentally more seasoned piece of the vagus nerve to endure. This is particularly the situation in circumstances such are reality compromising in which there will never be a way out. The dorsal vagal neural pathway is likewise part of the parasympathetic nervous system; in any case, this time immobilization turns into a guarded reaction. Ordinarily, this is alluded to as the "blackout" reaction. Some of the time, one can actually black out on the grounds that the dorsal vagal pathway diminishes blood stream to the brain. Shy of blacking out, this guarded pathway can prompt manifestations, for example, unsteadiness, queasiness, or exhaustion all side effects of separation.

Your physiology holds the recollections of injury as well as holds a significant key to recuperation. The Polyvagal theory guides us to another vital aspect for recuperating... your ability to connect with the social nervous system. You can encourage the strength of your social nervous system by creating careful attention to your body sensations, for example, your pulse or breath. This encourages you to identify your very own indications of stress and permits you to react immediately—before the stress feels overpowering or out of your control.

Consider the following;

- **Practice Attention Control**. Practice concentrating on specific signals in your condition that advise you that you are protected at this point. Check out your room. Notice the light sifting through a window, a bit of craftsmanship on the divider, or how it feels to peruse this article. You can likewise tune in to a most loved bit of music, grasp an article, or notice the quieting fragrance of a basic oil.

- **Self-Compassion.** Develop self-sympathy for your side effects. Perceive the physiological, substantial premise of side effects and why you can't just consider your method for your injury responses.

- **Create Somatic Awareness.** Learn to carefully follow unobtrusive changes in your body sensations and pulse. Identify your very own indications of stress. This will enable you to react immediately before the stress begins to feel overpowering or out of your control. We call this remaining in the window of resilience.

Conclusion

Thank you for making it through to the end of this volume on the *Vagus Nerve*. We hope it was informative and able to provide you with all of the tools you need to achieve your goals of improving your understanding of this important topic.

Please take the time to go over any part of this book which you feel is particularly important or relevant for you. Also, the information we have provided to help you improve your overall health and wellbeing. It is important for you to find a balance that can lead you to a better quality of life.

Indeed, the knowledge we have discussed in this book may be of benefit to you, or any one of your loved ones. So do take the time to get as much as you can out of this book. We are sure that you will not be disappointed in the results you can get from taking care of the vagus nerve. Plus, the information we have presented here will lead you to a better life, both physically and mentally.

We hope you will find plenty of benefits from the information we have distilled as a result of years and years of research and study.

Thank you once again for reading this book. See you at the next one!

www.ingramcontent.com/pod-product-compliance
Lightning Source LLC
Chambersburg PA
CBHW070712250726
48662CB00001B/379